Preparing for Interprofessional Teaching
Theory and practice

Preparing for Interprofessional Teaching

THEORY AND PRACTICE

Edited by

Elizabeth Howkins
Honorary Fellow, University of Reading
PIPE Project Lead

and

Julia Bray
Specialist Nurse Child Protection
Berkshire East PCT
PIPE Project Director

Foreword by
Hugh Barr
President, CAIPE
Professor Emeritus in Interprofessional Education
University of Westminster

Radcliffe Publishing
Oxford • New York

Radcliffe Publishing Ltd
18 Marcham Road
Abingdon
Oxon OX14 1AA
United Kingdom

www.radcliffe-oxford.com
Electronic catalogue and worldwide online ordering facility.

British Library Cataloguing in Publication Data

A catalogue record for this book is available from the British Library.

ISBN-13: 978 1 84619 098 8

Typeset by Phoenix Photosetting, Chatham, Kent
Printed and bound by Hobbs the Printers Ltd, Totton, Hampshire

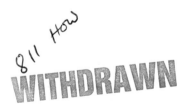

Contents

Foreword

More than a PIPE dream

Early writing about interprofessional education was inspired by the singleness of purpose and unswerving certainty of its pioneers, intent upon winning hearts and minds for the cause that they espoused. It would be hard to imagine the progress made during the early years had it not been for their inspiration. That progress prompted calls for closer scrutiny to convince employers, professions, pressure groups, universities, commissioners, regulators and government itself that inter-professional education will deliver what its exponents claimed. That is the challenge to which the new generation of interprofessional educators is rising as they record and document their projects, expose them to critical review, and share their experience openly and honestly. Less evangelical and more critical than their forebears, they are painstakingly assembling the emerging evidence base.

So far, so good, but interprofessional education is only as effective as its teaching, as students are quick to point out. Enter PIPE, which for three years explored different ways in different programmes in different settings to facilitate interprofessional learning. 'Facilitation', for the PIPE team, is not as a gratuitous addition to an already jargon-ridden vocabulary, but captures the distinctive qualities that engender dialogue and mutual learning between students from different professions to modify reciprocal attitudes and behaviour, heighten awareness of self and others, and cultivate co-working.

Readers in search of topical tips, techniques and quick fixes look elsewhere! Read on and you will find approaches, frameworks, models and theories to help you to understand interprofessional facilitation in all its complexity. Then, but only then, may you enjoy the liberation which is interprofessional learning to the full, for students and facilitator alike

Happily, PIPE was more than just another short-lived, locally-based interprofessional project whose experience was lost when funds ran dry. Evaluation was built in from the outset with the clear intention that lessons learned would be published, exposed to peer-review and accessible to others. This book is the outcome.

Its publication coincides with growing commitment to the improvement of interprofessional teaching and learning backed, like PIPE, by the Higher Education

Funding Council for England. The Higher Education Academy is in the forefront of these developments, working through three of its teaching and learning centres and complemented by many of the Centres of Excellence in Teaching and Learning (CETLs). The Centre for the Advancement of Interprofessional Education (CAIPE), to my pleasure, is working with former members of the PIPE team to update its rolling programme of workshops for those who will prepare and sustain the next generation of facilitators.

This book will reinforce all those endeavours. More than that, it will be an indispensable resource wherever, at home and abroad, universities and service agencies are intent upon building up a cadre of facilitators upon whose sensitivity and skill, establishing and maintaining the quality and credibility of interprofessional education depends.

Hugh Barr
President, CAIPE
Professor Emeritus in Interprofessional Education
University of Westminster
October 2007

Preface

Interprofessional education is an essential process for improving collaborative practice and the quality of patient/client care. Collaborative practice in the form of teamwork needs nurturing and supporting if it is to achieve its full potential to improve the health and well being of patients and service users. An opportunity to evaluate the teaching of interprofessional education and to use this evidence to examine and promote improvements in the quality of teaching interprofessional education was made possible through the PIPE project (Promoting Interprofessional Education), on which this book is based.

The book will address teaching interprofessional education from a variety of perspectives, offer some answers and raise many questions. It also provides a welcome addition to the growing body of knowledge that seeks to promote and improve the evidence base for interprofessional education. It does not intend to offer a 'how to do it teacher manual for interprofessional teaching and learning', nor an application of theory to practice. It does however, offer theories, frameworks and models of teaching interprofessional education (IPE) which we hope will make a contribution to the complex theoretical field of IPE. The PIPE team acknowledge that there are no simple solutions or one theory for IPE, but by using the evidence from the PIPE research project we expect to develop the thinking of both theory and practice for teachers involved in IPE. This book should help teachers to further understand their practice, clarify complex areas and to build their own theories of teaching interprofessional education.

The background to the PIPE project, some factual and historical details can be found in Appendix 1.

The main aims of the book are:

- to provide a critical exploration of practice issues relating to teacher preparation for interprofessional learning
- to propose frameworks for interprofessional learning and teaching
- to contribute to the emerging evidence base of teacher/facilitator preparation for interprofessional learning.

We hope that this book will be read by both teachers and practitioners working with health and social care professionals. It should provide the reader with a

Acknowledgements

The journey of the PIPE project and the production of this book has been helped in many ways and by many people. The contributions and continued support from these people has meant the PIPE project was able to achieve its goals. We are particularly grateful to Ann Ewens and Julie Hughes for spotting an opportunity to secure funding, setting up the project team and getting the consortium together.

We would also like to pay thanks to all members of our hard working steering group. This group made inter-organisational collaboration a reality, gave the project credibility and support at a senior level. The efficiency of the steering group was greatly assisted by its excellent chair, Professor Ginny Gibson, Director of Teaching and Learning at the University of Reading.

The project had four schemes which ran throughout its life; each of these was led by a scheme leader heading up a group of people who gave their time and expertise well beyond any requirements and/or expectations. To all of the scheme leaders and the group members we extend our heartfelt thanks.

The evaluation of the project was an essential requirement and to this, we are grateful for the expertise, support and commitment from our evaluator Dr Marilyn Hammick. Although many more people could be named for all their work over the project and preparation of the book, we would like to pay a special tribute to the two PIPE project directors, Ann Ewens in the first year and Julia Bray for the rest of the project's life. They both brought an element of enthusiasm, determination and excellent organisation to the project which ensured that it stayed on track and remained financially viable.

As with all large projects the time given by the PIPE team has been on the margins of their already heavy workloads, encroaching on family life, friends and social activities.

We want to end by saying a really big thank you to our husbands, partners, children and close friends for supporting and encouraging us to carry out this work.

List of abbreviations

BCUC	Buckinghamshire Chiltern University College
CAIPE	Centre for the Advancement of Interprofessional Practice and Education, UK
DoH	Department of Health
FDLT	Fund for the Development of Teaching and Learning (part of HEFC)
GP	General practitioner
HEFC	Higher Education Funding Council
HEI	Higher education institution
IL	Interdisciplinary learning
IPE	Interprofessional education
IPL	Interprofessional learning
JET	Joint evaluation team
LTSN	Learning and Teaching Support Network
MA	Higher degree qualification of Master of Arts
MD	Multidisciplinary
MP	Multiprofessional learning
MSc	Higher degree qualification of Master of Science
NHS	National Health Service
OBU	Oxford Brookes University
OPGMDE	Oxford Postgraduate Medical Deanery for Education
QAA	Quality Assurance Agency
PIPE	Promoting Interprofessional Education
PCT	Primary care trust
PHCT	Primary healthcare team
RAE	Research assessment exercise
SHA	Strategic Health Authority
SL	Shared learning
TVU	Thames Valley University
TSD	Training and Service Development Agency
UO	University of Oxford
UR	University of Reading
UK	United Kingdom
WHO	World Health Organisation

Glossary

Collaboration is an active ongoing partnership based on sharing, cooperation and coordination in order to solve problems and provide a service, often between people from very different backgrounds.

Continuing professional development is learning undertaken after initial qualification in order to maintain competence and develop professional capability.

Curriculum includes all the aspects that contribute to the learning: aims, content, mode of delivery, assessment, evaluation.

Facilitator is someone who embraces the notion of dialogue, is self aware, learns with the group but is able to provide the appropriate learning resources and create an environment for effective interprofessional education.

Interdisciplinary learning (IL) involves integrating the perspective of two or more professionals, by organising the education around a specific discipline, where each discipline examines the basis of their knowledge. (CAIPE (Centre for Advancement for Interprofessional Education) definition in Vanclay 1997).

Interprofessional education (IPE) Occasions when two or more professionals learn with, from and about each other together to improve collaboration and the quality of care (CAIPE 2007).

Interprofessional learning (IPL) a process in which different professionals learn from each other through interaction to develop collaborative practice. This may be in a formal education setting or opportunistically in the workplace.

Multidisciplinary (MD) involves bringing professionals with different perspectives together in order to provide a wider understanding of a particular problem.

Multiprofessional education (MP) describes a process by which a group of health-related professions with different educational backgrounds learn side by side for whatever reason.

Reflective learning is the ability to use reflection to make sense of an experience, to be able to verbalise thoughts, share with others and learn from the experience.

Shared learning (SL), a common term used to describe professional groups learning together.

Staff development continued professional development of staff through activities to enhance their knowledge and skills and change attitudes. It is sometimes referred to as faculty development in higher education.

Steering group is a group of people who support and advise a project.

Teacher. The PIPE team sees the teacher as part of the more formal structured delivery of education but they do acknowledge that the term facilitator and teacher are often interchanged.

Teamwork. A process whereby a group of people work together with a common goal.

Uniprofessional education is where members of a single profession learn together.

CHAPTER 1

Perspectives of interprofessional learning and teaching

ELIZABETH HOWKINS

Introduction

Over the past 30 years interprofessional education has gradually gained credibility as a way to increase and sustain collaborative practice between health and social care professionals. It is acknowledged that interprofessional education is challenging, but with careful planning and the appropriate use of teaching and learning approaches, it is possible. It is not, however, sufficient simply to place professionals together at certain stages in their careers and hope that they will learn to work together. Delivery of health and social care in the twenty-first century depends on multiprofessional approaches to complex health and social care problems. But professionals do need help and support to learn from, with and about each other to be able to provide collaborative care. Well-organised and well-taught interprofessional education programmes have to be put in place to prepare professionals for collaborative practice, both in college and in the workplace. What 'well-organised and well-taught' actually means for the teachers of interprofessional education will be discussed and explored in this book.

The timing of when to include interprofessional into the career of any health and social care professional has caused much debate and discussion.[1,2] Is it better to start in the pre-qualifying period with the hope of avoiding the development of negative professional stereotypes[3] or wait until after qualification when the professional should feel more confident in their role? Or can the two be amalgamated to incorporate all stages of professional development? Miller *et al*[1] proposed a useful model of interprofessional development which takes in the whole of the professional career, starting with the student, then the newly-qualified professional and ending with the professional leader stage. The various stages in the model include classroom, clinical and practice settings. Miller[1] does stress that to achieve a successful approach to interprofessional education all the interested parties, such as higher education institutions, health trusts, hospitals and social care have to be committed to working together with agreed outcomes to improve collaborative work.

The challenge for the PIPE team was to explore and find evidence about the kinds of teaching skills and methods used to promote interprofessional education (IPE) in the classroom and practical settings. A particular aim was to be able to provide evidence of the knowledge and skills needed by those preparing teachers for IPE. Much has been written about the barriers, the problems and the type of learning experience required to promote interprofessional education[4,5] but very little about the skills and knowledge needed on how to teach interprofessional groups. The focus of the PIPE project was to explore and research the teaching of IPE with the aim that by improving the quality of teaching in the learning environments there is a greater likelihood of achieving effective interprofessional work.

This first chapter places the project activities in the context of interprofessional education and provides a framework for the book. The chapter is divided into four sections.

- Section one: working definitions of interprofessional education, interprofessional learning and multiprofessional education.
- Section two: the need to improve interprofessional education teaching.
- Section three: aspects of the learning process for interprofessional education.
- Section four: aspects of teaching interprofessional education.

Section one: working definitions of interprofessional education, interprofessional learning and multiprofessional education

The PIPE team were well aware of the ongoing confusion with regard to the use of words and varying definitions relating to interprofessional education (IPE) and therefore intended to start by addressing some of the key issues over terminology and produce some working definitions, which will be used throughout the book and can be found in the glossary.

With the growth of interprofessional education, the necessity to have a clear understanding of what it entails has become evident, but as Barr argues, almost impossible. He describes the field[6] as a 'semantic quagmire where terms are used interchangeably or with seemingly precise but strictly private meanings'. Examples include, multidisciplinary, interdisciplinary, multiprofessional, shared learning and integrated learning; it is not difficult to see why this should arise. It is not the intention here to define or debate this myriad of definitions but only to address interprofessional education, interprofessional learning and multiprofessional education.

Until the 1990s, 'shared learning' was the common term used to describe professional groups learning together, but as Ewens[7] argues, from the mid-1980s a debate was taking place regarding a more precise definition. The term 'interprofessional education (IPE)' was gradually adopted, describing events where two or more professional groups learn together with the aim of promoting collaborative practice. The notion of aiming to promote collaborative practice is an essential aspect of any definition, because without it there would be 'no greater commitment than sitting students in the same classroom'.[7]

A survey of IPE initiatives[8] developed by the Centre for the Advancement of Interprofessional Education (CAIPE) produced a working definition of IPE using three criteria:

- the primary objective of the event is educational
- it involves participants of two or more selected professional groups
- participants are learning together within a multidisciplinary context.

But what was missing from this definition was the degree of learning and change as a result of the IPE experience.[9] Interprofessional education includes interaction from the participants to change their ways of knowing and understanding with the explicit aim of promoting interprofessional collaboration and improving the quality of care. The three important aspects of any definition of interprofessional education should incorporate the patient/client centred perspective along with collaborative practice and change of behaviour as a result of learning.

The term 'multiprofessional education' is often used interchangeably with interprofessional education particularly in its international usage. The World Health Organisation[10] uses the term 'multiprofessional education' and describes it as:

> The process by which a group of students from health-related occupations with different educational backgrounds learn together during certain periods of their education, with interaction as an important goal they collaborate in providing promotive, preventative, curative, rehabilitative and other health-related services.

Many countries use the term 'interprofessional education' and address collaboration and the patient perspective, such as the Australian Health Department which defines interprofessional education as:

> A collaborative, interdisciplinary education and learning process designed to produce effective, multidisciplinary patient-centred care.[11]

But the one definition that seems clearer, more manageable and closer to the focus of our project is the CAIPE definition of interprofessional education:[12]

> Occasions when two or more professions learn with, from and about each other to improve collaboration and the quality of care.

The PIPE project team embrace the CAIPE definition of interprofessional education and intend to be more specific, using the term 'interprofessional learning (IPL)' where appropriate. The rationale for this is that learning is placed at the centre of the process and reinforces the notion that interprofessional learning takes place in everyday situations in the workplace, as well as in planned programmes of interprofessional education. The use of the phrase 'interprofessional learning' is therefore understood to be an outcome of interprofessional education and it is 'learning that arises from interaction between two or more professions'.[13]

Having clarified the potential confusion over the terminology associated with professionals learning together, produced a very brief working definition of interprofessional education, interprofessional learning and multiprofessional education, the next section will address the original PIPE problem of 'why teaching for interprofessional learning needs to be improved.'

Section two: the need to improve interprofessional education teaching

In today's society and across the world there are increasing demands placed on the work and resources of health and social care professionals. These demands result from an ageing population, poverty, increasing technological advances and higher expectations of healthcare from the population. The complex issues of health and social care means that professionals must work together to deliver a quality service. Government policy in the UK in recent years has had a common theme:[14,15,16,17]

■ the need for better teamwork at all levels of health and social care services
■ the need for integrated care based on partnership
■ greater coordination and cooperation between the statutory and voluntary agencies.

But with later government policies another theme was added, that of patient-focused care.[18] This involved a huge culture shift from a paternalistic approach to one of partnership with the client/patient and carer, an approach which lent itself to collaborative work. To encourage and promote effective collaboration was an ambitious goal set by the government to establish working partnerships between services.[5] The challenge has been to find ways to encourage, promote and sustain interagency collaboration. In the UK, initiatives have taken place at local, regional and international level.[19] In addition, a recent Department of Health (DoH) document requires health and social care services to provide effective interprofessional education (IPE) both in the workplace and in undergraduate programmes in higher education institutes.[20] In light of this, interprofessional education is increasingly recognised as an effective way forward as a workable strategy for its importance in promoting partnership and shared learning.[21]

The rationale that interprofessional education promotes collaboration is based on the understanding that, by learning together, professionals have an opportunity to understand both their own role and those of others, to spend time exploring each other's belief and value systems and to share their expertise and knowledge. The argument then follows that by learning together, collaborative skills should be learnt, communication streamlined and ultimately patient/client care improved.[22]

However, interprofessional education is not an easy option. Professionals are trained and educated in their own disciplines, learning their own unique and specialist knowledge for their chosen profession. So, although each profession is well equipped for its singular contribution, they find their 'educational preparation a total mismatch for the complex, interactive world into which they graduate and practice'.[23] Consequently, the question of how to achieve effective interprofessional learning has exercised the minds of clinicians, practitioners, managers, academics and their respective professional and statutory bodies.[24] This wider debate will not be explored here, but only used to flag up to readers the one aspect the PIPE team intend to address, which is the preparation of teachers for interprofessional learning.

Although there are strong policy initiatives driving interprofessional education, up to now there has been little evidence of improved patient/client outcomes. The starting point must be the patient/client health and social care needs. There is also a commonsense approach that patients/clients do not want fragmented care and expect their professionals to be working effectively as a team. Individual health needs do not respect organisational boundaries, and neither do people want to fight their way through communication and organisation barriers to access care.[25] Educational initiatives that help foster mutual respect, understanding of roles and working as a team are therefore needed. But does this actually lead to better patient/client care? The first evidence of positive outcomes from both the patient/client and professional perspective was published in 2005 by Barr *et al.*[26] The work was the culmination of a systematic review of interprofessional education in health and social care. The systematic review team examined 107 high quality published evaluations of interprofessional education in health and social care. The findings from the review are extensive and build on many of the arguments and assumptions made about interprofessional education. Some evidence for three interprofessional education outcomes were reported in the study.

The areas are:
1 creates positive interaction between professionals
2 encourages collaboration between professions
3 improves patient/client care.

The authors[26] of the systematic review make no claim to 'expect a dramatic breakthrough in establishing the evidence base for interprofessional education', but do offer their work as a significant starting point for further rigorous studies.

The underpinning question at the start of this section was: why is there a need to improve IPE teaching and how might IPL outcomes be affected? So far the background literature to this question has been explored and discussed now the specific question will be addressed. In early meetings of the PIPE project, the team heard from teachers that they often felt ill prepared for their job of facilitating IPE groups and stated that they found the role difficult and were sometimes left feeling that the session was counter productive to the aims of IPE. One evaluation of a large scale health and social care undergraduate multiprofessional programme, the Joint Universities Multiprofessional Project (JUMP)[27] showed that the outcome of the learning experience did depend on the quality of facilitation skills and also that facilitation skills were often assumed, but not always present. Reeves *et al*[28] writing about an innovative interprofessional learning scheme on a ward in a London hospital, found that facilitation of interprofessional groups can be particularly demanding. Two of the same authors[2] describe a model of learning and teaching, and then go on to make the observation that 'poor facilitation of a collaborative learning experience is not only disappointing to learners; it can undermine their commitment to the value of working collaboratively'.

In a research study carried out by Mhaolrunaigh and Clifford[29] to evaluate the preparation of teachers for shared learning programmes, it was found that there was a need to prepare teachers to facilitate learning, but the type of preparation was not so clear cut. More recent work by Camsooksai[30] examining the role of the lecturer practitioner in interprofessional education highlighted the need for skilled committed IPE facilitators, a message reinforced by many other writers.[13,31]

In conclusion, there is a need to improve the quality of IPL teaching in order to ensure that all the resources, planning and organisation already going into IPL programmes have a much higher chance of a successful outcome for both the student and, in the long term, the patient/client. Teaching IPL is difficult, people are often ill-prepared and the sort of preparation needed is not yet clear. The next section introduces key concepts and perspectives on the learning process needed for interprofessional education.

Section three: aspects of the learning process for interprofessional education

> Occasions when two or more professions learn with, from and about each other to improve collaboration and the quality of care.[12]

In this definition there is an implication that learning must be interactive, that there should be a change of behaviour to improve collaborative practice and that the patient/client should benefit. But how this learning should take place, between whom and to what ends raises an important question for IPL.[32] The simple answer is, in a multitude of ways, in many settings, but not necessarily planned IPL sessions, which may or may not always be with other professionals. Two scenarios are given here to help to illustrate this point (*see* Boxes 1.1 and 1.2).

In the first scenario unrealistic aims for IPL had been set alongside too full a programme, but more importantly there was a failure to use the principles of interprofessional education and ensure that the appropriate teaching methods were employed. Whereas in scenario two, the interactive nature of the teaching session, and the use of the carers' real stories created a powerful and personal session which met IPL outcomes, although there were only members of one profession present. The boundary between interprofessional, multiprofessional and uniprofessional education may be clear, but operationally it is blurred and permeable.[26] The fact that IPL can develop in many ways and is not always planned

BOX 1.1 Scenario one

An IPL session with social workers, police, nurses and doctors.

An IPL session was set up with social workers, police, nurses and doctors to address local issues on the common assessment framework for child protection. It took place in the workplace, was not assessed, was compulsory and was part of continuing professional development. The session was full of new factual information and policy issues, no time was given to learning about other's roles, and the group did not have the opportunity to take away some strategies to improve future collaborative work. The evaluation indicated that the participants had learnt some of the new facts and policies but had found it a waste of time being with other professionals. They did not find the discussion about other professions either relevant to them or of any interest to them. The opportunity to use this time for professionals to learn more about each other, how they could communicate better and work together to make some joint decisions was not realised and it was an opportunity lost.

BOX 1.2 Scenario two

An undergraduate medical student session on working with carers in palliative care.

The session was set up with one set of professionals, medical students. For pragmatic reasons, at the time of development of these sessions, it was not possible to incorporate students from other professional groups. However, looking at the impact of interprofessional teamworking was one of the objectives of the workshop. Carers took part in the classroom education session. This meant that the medical students were exposed to real stories of good and poor teamwork. They also heard the carers' frustration when the service was experienced as fragmented and delight when it appeared to pull together. The medical students showed in their evaluation that they had changed their behaviour in relation to collaborative work because they really could empathise with the patient/carer perspective. For example, they realised the importance of communicating with the carers as well as the patients and recognised the exhaustion and isolation that carers experience. They also appreciated the importance of each professional's role in the whole picture and the necessity for good communication between professionals as well as with patients and their families.

must be seen as an opportunity and one that was found to be significant in the PIPE project.

However, IPL is more effective when the principles of interprofessional education are used in the planning and teaching process, whether the event takes place in the classroom, practice or other workplace venue. This chapter sets out a framework of the principles of interprofessional education,[26] whereas the following chapters discuss IPL teaching and learning strategies, characteristics, theories, models and influencing policies in detail.

Principles of interprofessional education

Collaborative learning: the ideal is that professions should develop mutual respect for one another, be able to value each other's contribution and learn ways to work together in practice. It is an approach encouraged by teachers but tribalism is never far away and dealing with professional rivalry is part of IPE teaching. Dealing with the damaging stereoptypes and making explicit some hidden agendas have to form part of the learning process.

Egalitarian learning: the aim in IPE is that everyone should learn from a level playing field. However, inequalities remain and are an inevitable part of professionalisation. It is the teaching process that has to deal with differences of status and power so that they do not interfere with the learning process.

Group directed learning: 'this comes into play when participants carry out collective responsibility for group assignments.'[26] In any professional group activity individuals can manage by making their own decisions or having their own goals, but when this has to be agreed with the group and the group have to develop strategies that actually work, then significant group learning is both challenged and realised.

Experiential learning: involves the participation in a process of direct experience using aspects from real life, which are patient/client centred, employing self-directed activities throughout, so that students learn with, from and about each other. By definition this must be interactive learning.

Reflective learning: the ability to use reflection in a group session means that the students make sense of their experience, they can verbalise their thoughts, share them with others and learn from their experience. Schon[33,34,35] has written extensively on reflective learning, in particular, distinguishing between reflection in action, where a quick decision is made, to reflection on action which involves time and support to learn from the experience.

In a study carried out by Wee and her colleagues[36] using workshops to share knowledge and learning between a range of professional disciplines, an interesting and useful approach to reflection was described. Professional reflection can be like looking in a mirror, describing what you see, i.e. the professional work. But taking this analogy a little further, Wee goes on to use the idea of a hairdressers' three-way mirror where you are shown views of yourself you do not normally see and maybe in reality you do not want to see. The group of participants in the workshop can create this three-way mirror reflection by discussing their practice with the group in a safe secure learning environment.

Applied learning: 'relates the content and experience of interprofessional education to collaborative practice.'[26] It is about how to plan, organise and structure educational sessions that should overcome potential barriers and develop strategies that are known to be effective to enhance interprofessional learning outcomes. The process on which the experience is founded is consistent with adult learning principles, such as students bringing their own experience to the learning situation thus providing a rich learning resource; that the learning experience should be authentic and based on real life issues and that the adult student is self-directing.[37,38]

The challenge to the teacher of interprofessional learning is to provide the educational experience in the appropriate environment which incorporates the above principles of interprofessional education.

Section four: aspects of teaching interprofessional education

The role of an interprofessional education teacher is both challenging and demanding. Planning, organising and delivering IPL sessions requires creativity and confidence but above all the teacher has to become aware of self and use of self. Research into interprofessional education has consistently focused on the learner's perspective; such as how they learn, what are the barriers and what helps learning, but research studies have not addressed the teacher perspective. Various researchers[2,31,39] have called for the need for specific preparation of teachers for IPL, noting that it does require more in-depth skills than uniprofessional teaching. In the UK where there have been large undergraduate health and social care educational programmes, (JUMP project in North West London workforce and Southampton University, New Generation project)[27,40] special facilitator workshops have been set up as part of the ongoing programme. Acquiring the skills and gaining the confidence to facilitate IPL groups is not an easy option. One of the first European countries committed to interprofessional education (referred to as multiprofessional education) was Norway. They used an education approach known as 'scenario-based problem solving'. They found that teaching staff felt deskilled and demotivated as they were only expected to facilitate learning, not to impart their knowledge of their specialist subject.[1] IPL teaching requires a different approach from teaching in a didactic manner to a more facilitative style and one where the teacher also becomes the learner. It is this change of approach from formal teaching to a facilitative teaching style that encompasses much of the work of the PIPE project. A brief exploration of teacher as facilitator will follow to set the context of how the term will be used throughout the book.

Over the years the role of the teacher has constantly evolved and changed. No longer is the teacher the font of all wisdom, 'knowledge is now too vast to be contained'.[41] Sarles, in his book *Teaching as Dialogue*,[41] goes on to argue that a teacher needs to enter into a dialogue with their students. Dialogue is for Sarles an exploration, mode of search and critical inquiry enabling and inviting students to think. Sarles draws on the work of Freire[42,43] where he talks about building on relationships of vulnerability and power to overcome abuse and oppression. The role of the teacher/facilitator must be to use dialogue with students to explore learnt behaviour and be able to inspire them to learn and change. During the process of professional socialisation damaging stereotypes of other professions are learnt and then become part of every day professional behaviour. An essential stage therefore, of interprofessional education is to help the participants to explore these damaging stereotypes, understand each other's professional view and thus avoid further perpetuation of these in the workplace.

Although Freire's work was with an adult literacy programme in Brazil it does offer a theoretical perspective which helps to frame the work of an IPL facilitator.[44] The recognition that people can be constrained and oppressed by their life world but unable to see it, unaware of how it influences them and unable to make changes was the starting point for Freire's concept 'conscientisation'. He used the term to describe the development of critical awareness, a process where learners can step outside forces that lead them to conformity and seek to liberate thought processes. Conscientisation or 'awareness raising' is an open-ended learning process carried out through group dialogue. The role of the group leader for Freire was that of facilitator, someone who has an open mind and does not lecture. The qualities of the leader were to be critical, encouraging, listening, not interrupting, able to speak their own thoughts and not just accept, but also to analyse.

Health and social care professionals come to IPL sessions with their own beliefs and values, stereotypes of other professions and their own learning styles. The professional socialisation process and the pre-conceived views about IPL mean that there are very powerful influences and constraints in place for any IPL session. Many people may also feel disempowered in a mixed professional group. Understanding the process of dialogue and the facilitator role to develop critical awareness has many similarities to the process of facilitation under review in this book. In IPL and in the work of Freire the facilitation process must address sensitive issues such as race, gender, beliefs and politics. Freire regards it as essential to reflect on the meanings and any disjuncture these may cause to the group.

A particular strength of Freire's work is the link between education, the person and political agendas. A diagramatic representation of this is shown in Chapter 2 through the use of the Illeris Tension Triangle.[45]

Using Freire's work on group facilitation and identifying what this means for the PIPE project is the next step. A facilitator is someone who makes it easy to learn, to provide opportunities to learn and does not just give out information or teach in a didactic manner. It is also a means of encouraging and supporting individuals and groups to find their most effective way of learning. It is, to use

Freire's words about empowering people to believe in themselves, to become active learners rather than passive.[46]

In this book, the term 'facilitator' will be used to mean someone who embraces the notion of dialogue, is self aware, learns with the group but is also able to provide the appropriate learning resources and create an environment for effective interprofessional learning. The PIPE team see the teacher as part of the more formal structured delivery of education but we do acknowledge that the terms are often interchanged.

It is not the intention here to discuss the many styles of facilitation or the skills of facilitation used with groupwork, but only to examine our use of the term 'facilitation' and provide a working definition. The reader is recommended to many excellent books on facilitation such as: Bee and Bee,[47] Hogan,[48] and Hunter et al.[49] One writer that has proved particularly useful in our work is John Heron, formerly head of the Human Potential Resources Group at the University of Surrey and author of the *Complete Facilitator's Handbook*.[50] His six dimensional models provide a framework which follows a series of steps:

1 the operating dimension
2 the planning dimension
3 the confronting dimension
4 the meaning dimension
5 the valuing dimension
6 the feeling dimension.

All these dimensions are needed and cannot be ignored, Heron writes that they 'interweave and overlap, but are mutually supportive'.[51] The significance to our work is the importance of the feeling or emotional aspects of learning; an area so often ignored in most professional education.

At the beginning of the PIPE study it was evident from examples brought from practice that there was a lack of clarity over the role of trainer and facilitator which often meant that the learning process for collaborative practice was lost. The facilitator frequently had a dual role, that of trainer and facilitator but did not have the necessary skills of IPL facilitation. As a result the group learnt about the subject but the experience of interprofessional learning was poor or non existent as shown in scenario one (*see* Box 1.1).

Before leaving this discussion on the facilitator it is necessary to point out that there are many other uses of the word 'facilitator' which cause misunderstanding and confusion. For example, a facilitator can be someone who has managerial responsibilities, who holds a job description aimed at changing the way people work, so in essence they are change agents or managers. Another role that added to the confusion is that of practice facilitator, this is someone with a remit to organise aspects of education practice, plan practice placements, run study days, and act as mentor and/or supervisor to a range of professionals. Also the word 'facilitator' is used very loosely to mean anyone who organises training sessions or even someone who has a chairing role at meetings.

Conclusion

Teachers are frequently ill prepared for teaching IPL and thus find the teaching experience both difficult and challenging. Much has been written about the barriers, the problems and the type of learning needed to promote IPL, but little about the process of teaching, the required skills and knowledge needed for effective IPL. The teacher of IPL has to provide the educational experience in the appropriate environment which incorporates the principles of IPL education.

The term interprofessional learning is used as it is more central to our work in the PIPE project on teacher improvement. The use of the word facilitator, rather than teacher is used as it reflects the importance of learning with and from the group and the need to be self aware.

The next chapter develops theories of learning and teaching, explores some of the challenges faced by facilitators of interprofessional learning at micro and macro level and discusses the value of the Tension Triangle developed by Illeris[45] as a potentially useful framework for lecturers, teachers and facilitators involved in IPL.

CHAPTER 2

A learning and teaching framework for interprofessional learning

KATY NEWELL-JONES AND MAGGIE LORD

To understand another's speech, it is not sufficient to understand his words – we must understand his thought. But even that is not enough – we must know his motivation.

Vygotsky[1]

Introduction

The focus of the PIPE project was for the preparation of health and social care professionals who had an educational role, to develop their understanding, skills and approaches to promoting interprofessional learning. The role of the practice educator, tutor, lecturer or facilitator is key in supporting interprofessional working practices, however, limited attention had previously been placed on how such people could best be prepared, it being assumed that their experience of working in health and social care would be sufficient.

The PIPE project consisted of four schemes which ran in parallel throughout the project. Each scheme explored the question:

How best do we develop educators with the skills, knowledge and attitude to promote interprofessional learning?

The context and specific focus in which the schemes' work took place included the following:

- a single Postgraduate Certificate in Medical Teaching programme primarily targeting general practitioners (GPs) (scheme one)
- four MSc/MA Education programmes in higher education institutions (HEIs), each with multiprofessional cohorts to varying degrees (scheme two)
- work-based practice education (scheme three)
- collaboration between programme teams from two HEIs, one involved only in undergraduate medical education and the other involved in the education and training of nurses, midwives and a range of other health and social care professionals, but not doctors (scheme four).

Although the context of each scheme differed, the challenges faced by lecturers, tutors, facilitators and teachers in developing effective approaches to promote interprofessional learning (IPL) were remarkably similar.

Effective IPL emphasises the importance of appropriate attention to development, delivery and evaluation. Educators in health and social care are invariably faced with a range of choices at each of these stages. They are expected and would like to be able to select, adapt and use a wide range of teaching strategies and choose appropriately from a plethora of 'useful' teaching techniques and interventions. Although lecturers and facilitators often seek 'hints and tips' to add to 'their toolkit', when asked to brainstorm different tools they have no difficulty in producing lengthy lists. The challenge appears to be which to select when and why, rather than identifying the options. Hence the PIPE team has sought to understand the complexity of IPL in the belief that this will lead to more informed decision making on the part of ourselves, and others, as educators. The discussions held throughout the PIPE project were helpful to the participants of all of the schemes but particularly to those whose institutions involved offered programmes at masters level in teaching and learning. In the same way as it was assumed that experienced practitioners could facilitate workplace interprofessional initiatives, there was a general assumption that interprofessional education sessions would be suitable for novice teachers as the content was perceived to be undemanding. Although the course teams did not believe this to be true, as there was a lack of evidence or framework to either support or contradict this general belief. While general learning theories are useful, a way of exploring such theories and determining their usefulness for preparing teachers for interprofessional learning was required.

This chapter begins by exploring some challenges of interprofessional teaching through the use of two brief scenarios drawn from experiences across the six institutions involved in PIPE and discussions with other health and social care professionals involved in IPL. This is followed by a discussion of the work of Knud Illeris[2,3,4,5] and his Tension Triangle as a model of understanding some of the tensions which lecturers, tutors, practice educators and teachers face when planning and facilitating IPL. The PIPE project team has found the work of Illeris[2,3,4,5] stimulating in making sense of the complexity of IPL and providing a framework within which to view a range of approaches to learning, together with the inherent tensions. The Tension Triangle allows for the positioning of programmes and events in relation to the cognitive, psychodynamic and the societal elements of the learning event and encourages practitioners to take this into account when selecting their approaches to learning and teaching. Illeris' work is explored in relation to IPL with reference to contact hypothesis and social identity theory.

The next part of the chapter integrates and applies the theory of IPL with the practice of teaching through discussion using the two scenarios. Finally, the chapter finishes with a range of points for consideration for lecturers, tutors and facilitators of IPL.

The challenges of interprofessional learning

Below are two scenarios constructed from discussion with professionals involved in interprofessional learning and which highlight many of the challenges faced by novice and experienced educators. They will be introduced briefly here, then discussed in more detail towards the end of the chapter in the context of the theoretical models introduced.

BOX 2.1 Scenario A

Interprofessional learning; a suitable role for a newly appointed lecturer?

A new lecturer is appointed to her first post in higher education. She comes with excellent clinical skills and some experience of teaching, usually focusing on the clear and coherent transfer of knowledge and acquisition of skills. She will undertake a teacher preparation course within her first two years. In her first semester she is asked to teach a number of sessions on modules where she brings specific subject expertise and also to contribute to undergraduate interprofessional modules where the content is generic and includes team work, leadership, transcultural care, inclusion and diversity and constructing a personal profile. She might even be told not to worry too much about the IPL module as the content is 'not very taxing' and the idea is to get people developing skills of interprofessional working practice.

In scenario A the new lecturer faces a complex set of challenges which might not become apparent until difficulties arise and she has an opportunity to understand the differences between the two radically different types of sessions she has been asked to teach. In order to be successful, she probably needs to adopt different approaches to teaching and learning for these two sessions, yet how does she decide which approaches to select?

BOX 2.2 Scenario B

Adopting the appropriate focus for interprofessional learning.

A social worker, respected for his work on child protection and a highly skilled educator, is invited to deliver a workshop for an interprofessional team. Difficulties in timetabling mean the session could either be one hour on the end of a team meeting, where most of the team will be present, or a longer session, with limited representation from the team. There are tensions within the team with different aspirations from the session. Some are expecting a focused up-date on legal aspects, aware of recent high profile cases in the media. Others feel that case review meetings could be more effective and would like the team to be communicating more effectively with each other. Yet others feel the child focus gets lost on occasions and would value extending their skills in working with parents and children.

In scenario B the social worker faces a range of challenges from planning through to the delivery of the session. He might have the skills as an educator to adopt a range of approaches to learning, from delivering an excellent, structured mini-lecture on the legal situation in respect of child protection to sensitively facilitating difficult discussions exploring areas of tension between professionals in teams. Again his challenge is to select which approach, or combination of approaches to adopt.

Illeris' framework

The scenarios outlined at the beginning of this chapter illustrate the complexity of decision-making facing tutors, lecturers and facilitators as they plan, deliver and evaluate interprofessional sessions. This complexity is widely recognised in the literature as is the search for theoretical frameworks within which to view IPL.[6] Complexity also emerged strongly from the focus group interviews with programme teams and students on MSc/MA education programmes engaged in the PIPE project, where the feeling of almost overwhelming complexity was matched with a search for clarity and definite answers. Although other frameworks and theories could be employed, it is the fact that Illeris can be used to explore complex and competing views and values in teaching and learning, and also accommodate them, that is its strength as an exploratory framework.

Novice and experienced educators in health and social care, undertaking programmes in learning and teaching, are often faced with an array of models of learning and teaching and face the challenge of selecting the appropriate approach to learning for any one context. These models are often introduced in chronological order which can imply sequential improvement and therefore the impression that the more recent models are most appropriate for current contexts. Newell-Jones[7] began exploring the use of Illeris' Tension Triangle[2,3,4,5] as an overarching framework within which to position different theoretical approaches to learning and to understand some of the tensions in IPL. Illeris' work has resonated through the PIPE project both in relation to understanding the choices facing tutors and lecturers and in exploring the emotive and societal dimension of interprofessional encounters, including identity defence and learning resistance. Like Sterling[8] who, in his Schumacher briefing 'Sustainable Education', nests educational systems within social, economic and cultural systems, Illeris[3,4] views education and learning as situated within a wider societal framework, illustrated by placing the Tension Triangle within an overall circle. The values base on which both Sterling and Illeris construct their models recognises the global interdependency of the twenty-first century, with a strong social justice agenda, additional factors which reflect the current thinking in learning and health and social care.

Building from a constructivist standpoint, Illeris bases his model (Figure 2.1) on two assumptions. Firstly that learning includes a dynamic combination of two processes; an internal process of acquisition at the level of the individual, of making sense of new knowledge and skills in the context of existing knowledge, and an external process of the learner interacting with the environment.[1]

The internal process of acquisition involves 'linking between new impulses and the results of prior learning'.[5(p83)] As such it is a highly individual process where the internal sense made by individuals with diverse backgrounds might be quite different, even though they participate in the same session, alongside one another. Learners from different professional backgrounds will come with different prior learning experiences and probably different concepts of effective learning. It is likely these differences will be evident even at the undergraduate level as they will usually be studying uniprofessional modules alongside any interprofessional modules. For example the emphasis on reflective learning is strong in nursing and midwifery;[9] the principles of adult learning are central to general practitioner (GP) training.[10]

When working with a diverse group, the highly individual nature of the process of the acquisition will inevitably lead to vast differences in the new sense which different participants make of their experiences. In Chapter 3, Bray explores the concept of the interprofessional group as a complex, diverse entity and the facilitation skills required to support learning in such a group.

The external process of interaction will depend on the opportunities to engage with others within the learning environment and also subsequent interactions. Through a process of dialogue learners adapt and modify their first interpretation of new learning and make sense of it in relation to other people. Within the IPL workplace there are a number of barriers to discussion, debate and collaborative learning including geographical distance, workload pressures, status

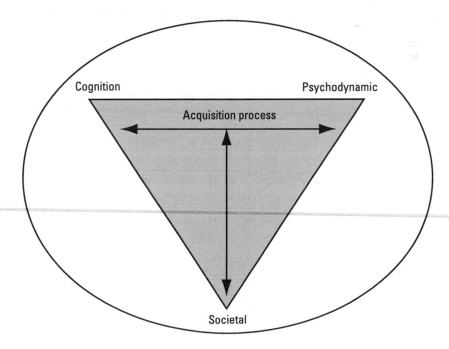

FIGURE 2.1 Illeris Tension Triangle (adapted from Illeris 2002).

and traditional patterns of communication. Sheppard, cited in Payne,[11] for example, describes differences in the focus on individual or collective responsibility for decision-making between GPs and social workers. Therefore, when promoting IPL, it is vital that it is not assumed that this process of interaction will automatically take place in the workplace but is a planned element of all learning activities.

Illeris' second assumption is that all learning events have elements of three dimensions:

1 cognitive, associated with the acquisition of knowledge and skills
2 psychodynamic, associated with motivation and emotion
3 societal, associated with communication and interaction with the outside world.[6]

One of the strengths of the Tension Triangle is that it is visually striking and can be used as a centrepiece for discussion drawing in theoretical frameworks from education and social science.

Traditionally, health and social care education has focused most strongly on the acquisition of knowledge and skills, i.e. located primarily in the cognitive corner. However, even learning a straightforward clinical procedure has a psychodynamic aspect. Motivation can be influenced by factors including the perceived value of the procedure, the tone of the educator and whether or not the learner will be assessed. Whether a particular learner is anxious or excited about learning is also likely to influence their learning. In an interprofessional context, professional identities and boundaries are quite likely to be challenged and the potential for emotional responses is considerable. Carpenter and Hewstone[12] recognise the negative and positive impact of emotions in interprofessional groups, for example anxiety of tensions and friendship between group members. Illeris places the cognitive and psychodynamic aspects of learning at different corners of his Tension Triangle, whereas Pettigrew[13] refers to the role of emotions in learning as one of four cognitive processes which mediate attitude change. Pettigrew's other three processes are more societal in nature and referred to below. Illeris uses the term 'identity defence'[5] to describe the situation when learning is hampered by the emotional response of identity being challenged. He describes occasions when redundant mature skilled workers struggling with their identity being stripped away from them, demonstrated emotional barriers to acquiring new skills and knowledge which would usually have been within their ability.[5] Similarly, where people perceive IPL as a process of breaking down professional boundaries, possibly leading to the generic healthcare worker or a cost-cutting exercise, the result might be identity defence which hinders the potential for positive outcomes from the learning event.

All learning also has a societal element, which in the case of IPL is recognised as being a central aspect, focusing on participants learning from and about each other. These crucial societal aspects of IPL are explored using contact theory[14] and social identity theory[15,16] in the Higher Education Academy Occasional Paper 7 theory-practice relationships in interprofessional education.[6] Carpenter and Hewstone[12] explore stereotyping using the concepts of in-groups, (those groups to which we feel an allegiance) and out-groups (those groups to which we do not feel we belong). The process of stereotyping results in the tendency to see in-groups as diverse, i.e. the members are viewed as having individual personalities, strengths and weaknesses, whereas out-groups are often perceived as homogenous, displaying common attributes which might be seen as highly positive, quaint, or more negatively as disruptive or abusive. Allport[17] reminds us that contact *per se* is not enough and that attention needs to be given to specific factors which support interaction, challenge and change. Pettigrew's[13] other three processes to mediate attitudinal change were firstly, providing opportunities for participants to learn about out-groups. This might have the effect of enlarging the in-group, or of challenging expectations and assumptions about out-group members. Secondly Pettigrew[13] recognised the value of the cognitive dissonance experienced when out-group members' behaviour is identified as different from the perceived stereotype and yet also seen as representative of the out-group. This dissonance might result in rejecting the new information and perceiving and valuing only behaviours which reinforce the stereotype. Alternatively, if the learning environment is safe and enabling, frameworks might be dismantled and new understandings formed. Finally, Pettigrew[13] recognises the value of 'intergroup contact' as providing an opportunity for individuals and group members to hear how they are perceived by others, in this instance other professionals.

One of the challenges which arise from Pettigrew's processes to mediate attitudinal change is for lecturers, tutors and facilitators to embrace and even encourage dissonance and tension. This needs to be accompanied by the skills to support participants through the process of understanding and learning from these situations. As health and social care practitioners the priority is often to create a learning environment where dissonance and discomfort is minimised. The lecturer might even see their role as moving swiftly away from conflict and tension, which might limit the opportunity for individuals and groups as a whole to explore differences and experience the dissonance which might lead to transformational learning.

Although the precise positions are contested, Illeris[2] maps the major theoretical approaches to working with groups and individuals within the Tension Triangle (Figure 2.2) with Piaget, Bandura, Kolb, Mezirow and Brookfield positioned to differing degrees in the cognitive corner, Freud and Rogers in the psychodynamic corner, and Marx and Bruner in the societal corner. Traditional approaches to learning are seen as focusing strongly on the cognitive aspects. The work of Rogers brought the emotive aspect of learning into focus and Jarvis, Bruner and Wenger have included a stronger societal element. We have added Allport[17] representing contact theory and social identity theory and also Freire[18] with his emphasis on the dialogical, collaborative nature of learning, being concerned with praxis, enhancing community and building social capital. Both Allport and Freire are located between the psychodynamic and societal corners.

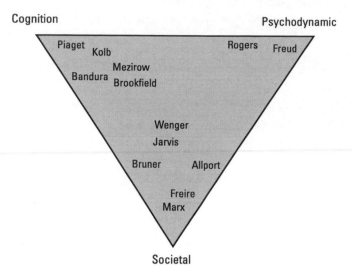

FIGURE 2.2 Illeris Tension Triangle (adapted from Illeris 2002).

As indicated, the explicit inclusion of the three dimensions is highly relevant to IPL. The focus of shared learning is of identifying content which is of value to two or more professional groups and bringing them together to learn alongside each other; a process which sits comfortably in the cognitive corner of the triangle. However, where IPL is seen as a process whereby two or more professionals engage in a process of learning with, from and about each other, the societal aspect of learning is placed at the centre of the process. The explicit recognition of tribalism within IPL is a strong reminder that the emotive element of learning possibly plays a stronger role in IPL than in uniprofessional learning. Hence when IPL focuses on learning with from and about other professionals, the appropriate model of learning could be argued to be positioned equidistant from the three corners, where Illeris[2] places Wenger's communities of practice.

Illeris[6] links the processes of making sense of new experiences to the learning descriptors of Nissen and others. He defines four kinds of learning; cumulation, assimilation, accommodation and transformation. Cumulative learning is where new knowledge is not located in relation to existing learning; assimilative learning involves primarily incorporation of new learning into existing frameworks which are then strengthened. Accommodative learning is where new understanding cannot be readily fitted into existing frameworks, which therefore need to be partially deconstructed and remodelled, a process which requires motivation and can be enormously challenging. Finally, transformational learning, which was originally described by Mezirow[19] is where fundamental underpinning values and concepts are challenged and restructuring often needs to take place, Illeris suggests, at the cognitive, emotive and societal levels.[5]

The intentions of IPL are often described in terms of challenging stereotypes and misconceptions. This would suggest that IPL focuses on accommodative and transformative learning, rather than cumulative and assimilative, especially at the post qualifying level where professional identities are well established. The description of transformational learning resonates with what people often describe as 'interprofessional-aha' moments, for example when a group or an individual realise that they have been viewing a certain situation through the lens of their own profession and that some of their strong judgements with which they previously felt very comfortable suddenly seem misplaced.

Applying the theory of IPL to teaching practice

Illeris' Tension Triangle provides a framework within which to debate the tensions faced by lecturers, tutors and facilitators working in interprofessional contexts. The framework recognises existing theories of learning and enables them to be positioned in relation to each other and in this chapter elements of contact theory and social identity theory have been woven into the debate. The Tension Triangle is firmly rooted in a constructivist approach to learning and teaching, with a tendency towards transformational learning. In other words, it assumes that the learner, in this case the health or social care educator, will be engaged in a process of making new sense of learning and teaching, challenging and sometimes rejecting previously held views and constructing their own personal perspective.

The way in which we have used Illeris, as a tool for educators to understand tensions and recognise choices, challenges the traditional view of teacher preparation as a process of acquiring a set of tools and the ability to select and apply the right tools for the task. The Illeris framework does not give definitive answers, nor in itself suggest strategies for facilitation but rather it can provide a framework within which to debate the issues and lead to more informed choices. As a model it requires a range of educational experience and knowledge on which to draw. It also requires the assumption that there are no definitive answers in terms of the selection of approaches to learning and teaching, rather the acceptance that different approaches will have different outcomes and that the role of the educator is to select between possible options in an informed manner. It may also have limited value where the preparation of health and social care educators is based on the presumption that the acquisition of new knowledge and skills should take precedence over the emotive or societal elements of learning.

Returning to the two scenarios at the beginning of the chapter, in the first scenario by positioning the learning outcomes of the two sessions within the Tension Triangle the lecturer will see that the two sessions are positioned very differently. The subject-based teaching is likely to have learning outcomes which are largely knowledge and skills and hence would be located primarily on the cognitive corner of the triangle. The session could be taught through a 'product' approach to learning, based on the lecturer as expert. At its most basic, the role of the lecturer is to be up-to-date with their own expertise and to provide a set of activities for the learners to acquire a range of knowledge and skills. As the new lecturers develop their expertise in learning and teaching they will hopefully adopt a range of participative approaches to learning which will greatly enhance the learning, but they can begin quite successfully from a model of learning based on lecturing, questions and answers and limited groupwork.

The interprofessional session, on the other hand, is likely to have learning outcomes which are more attitudinal and interactive in nature. Depending on the topic, they are more likely to be positioned away from the cognitive corner and more centrally in the Tension Triangle. There might be a number of divisions into sub-groups based on learners developing professional identities. Some of these sub-groups are likely to be making assumptions about each other based on stereotypes of professions which might be detrimental to effective groupwork and possibly poor professional practice in practice settings. This session therefore requires more of a process-based approach to learning. The role of the lecturer is not necessarily to be the provider of expert knowledge but to facilitate the group, providing them with an environment within which they can learn with, from and about other professionals. To do this they will need to establish a safe and trusting environment. If the topic is dealt with at a very superficial level, the group might be frustrated and disengaged. If the group explore differences between professions in depth, the group dynamics might be highly challenging with tribalism between professions in the form of defensiveness or aggression. When faced with such tensions, the new lecturer is likely, initially at least, to view the issues from the perspective of their own profession. The degree to which they are comfortable with tension and possible disagreement will also influence the extent to which they move the group constantly onto safer ground or whether they can support and encourage the group to explore tensions with the potential benefit of accommodative or transformative learning taking place. The greatest challenge for new lecturers can be recognising that they have both types of sessions in their portfolio of teaching and hence need to approach the preparation and delivery of each in a different way.

In the second scenario, the facilitator comes with their own professional background and perspective which informs their practice and provides them with a strong set of priorities and a specific values base which will overlap with, but differ to some extent from those of other professionals. Other members in the team might differ strongly from each other in their perspective. There may be a number of in-groups who communicate very little with each other on a regular basis and have strong expectations and assumptions of each other. There are also likely to be internal hierarchies in the team, based perhaps on professional status, or numerical dominance or other factors.

The length of the session and the membership of the group are strong factors in deciding the nature of the session. There is perhaps a tension between their preference which might be a session of two hours where tensions could be fully explored and the likelihood that this length of session will have limited representation.

The lecturer also needs to consider the factors which might attract various team members to commit to attending the session and these might be quite different from those which result in a successful session. Some individuals might only attend the session if their desire for specific knowledge are met. However, these same individuals might value a session where the outcomes include an increased awareness of the roles and responsibilities of team members and the revision of the structure of case review meetings. It is likely that the learning needs of individuals will need to be balanced with those of the team.

We opened this chapter with a quotation from Vygotsky[1] in which he places a high value on knowing the thoughts, and the motivation behind the words spoken by others in order to truly understand their speech. This links with recognising the psychodynamic element of learning and also the need for dialogue as an essential element of the learning process, i.e. a recognition that all three elements of learning are required for full understanding and exchange.

Points for teachers of IPL to consider

- The importance of understanding the context of the situation as fully as possible in advance. This includes the diversity within the group, different perspectives, different educational backgrounds and expectations, and the extent to which people within the group know each other and have had an opportunity to develop an understanding of each other's roles. In more complex groups (scenario B) this might also include understanding power and hierarchical relationships.
- The value of exploring where within Illeris' Tension Triangle the learning outcomes for each session are primarily located. Are they more concerned with the acquisition of new knowledge and skills (cognitive), or are they focused more on exploring attitudes and awareness (psychodynamic)? Or, are they concerned with participants engaging with each other and exploring relationships in practice (societal). If the learning outcomes are very diverse, decisions might need to be made about the primary focus for the session, or for specific parts of the session.
- Active selection of an approach, or approaches, to learning which matches the location of the intended learning outcomes will help create the appropriate learning environment. For example, if the learning intentions focus on participants learning with, from and about each other's roles, this will require an approach which relies on collaborative learning and develops a high level of trust. If the intention is to transmit knowledge, a more tutor-centred approach might be acceptable. A novice lecturer might need to identify one of two similar approaches for a session, whereas a more experienced facilitator will be able to adopt a range of styles appropriate to different aspects of a session with fluency.
- Participants' own previous experiences of learning will influence their expectations. If they are more familiar with sessions based on the acquisition of knowledge and skills, they will bring these expectations with them. Within an

interprofessional group, different groups might have very different expectations of a seminar or workshop.

■ Being explicit about the approach selected can help the participants to appreciate the nature of the intended session and to adjust some of their expectations. The importance of investing time in developing the appropriate learning environment is recognised in the literature and from the findings from the PIPE projects.

■ As lecturers or facilitators, self-awareness of our own feelings in relation to the content and the participants is important when facilitating complex diverse groups, especially around potentially emotive topics. Identity defence is not confined to the participants; lecturers and facilitators can be just as vulnerable. A novice lecturer might rely primarily on considering these issues in advance of a session, being aware of the issues and reflecting on them following the session. A more experienced facilitator will have developed their ability to reflect in action and to adapt their style as a result.

■ Lecturers and facilitators in interprofessional groups come with two or more identities; one stems from their own professional health or social care background and the other from their role as educator. When the professional identity of the lecturer dominates their interventions, this can leave the group without an effective facilitator, and with the lecturer using their powerful position to present the perspective of one professional group. This is also likely to trigger strong responses among participants.

■ Illeris' model recognises the highly individual nature of the learning process and the need for time to engage in the processes of acquisition and interaction. Recognising the value of the societal and emotional elements of learning and the creative role of dissonance in accommodative and transformational learning which are intended outcomes of interprofessional learning include challenging stereotypes and attitudinal change. This is the process of making sense of new experiences, often needing to adapt existing frameworks of knowledge, sometimes needing to reject existing frameworks and construct new ones. Where attitudes are challenged, learning defence behaviours might be triggered.

■ Recognising the value of the participants as a key learning resource in IPL. For the novice lecturer this might mean using the experiences and perspectives of participants in their professional practice as the source of material for discussion and debate. For the more experienced facilitator this might include negotiating the content and style of the session, responding to feedback at a micro and macro level and actively seeking evaluative comment on both the content and process of sessions.

Conclusions

An exploration of IPL in the light of the experiences of the PIPE project team and the work of Illeris[2,3,4,5] and others has led to a number of points for consideration for lecturers, tutors and facilitators involved in IPL. Although, many of these points are reflected elsewhere in the literature, the need for the lecturer or tutor to be aware of their own identities, as educator and health or social care professional, to develop the ability to select the focus on their role as educator and where appropriate, allow their professional identity to play a less dominant role, has not been explored to any great extent in the other IPL literature. The themes identified will be explored further in subsequent chapters, which both support and expand on the discussion in this chapter.

CHAPTER 3

Interprofessional facilitation skills and knowledge: evidence from a Delphi research survey

JULIA BRAY

Introduction

The previous chapter explored the challenges faced by teachers, lecturers and facilitators of interprofessional learning in health and social care. The discussion raises many of the tensions faced by professionals facilitating IPL groups and provides the Illeris framework[1] within which to consider the challenges but does not give answers on how to facilitate IPL groups. We continue here by exploring in depth the facilitation of IPL and the development of skills and teaching methods needed for the preparation of facilitators undertaking work-based learning. This is particularly important considering that a significant amount of IPL takes place in the workplace and that notwithstanding a plethora of government proposals, the evidence on the ground for effective interprofessional learning (IPL) initiatives in practice is varied.

This chapter outlines the research using a Delphi Survey,[2] where an expert panel of facilitators were selected throughout the UK in health and social care. The Delphi survey is a consensus method which is an iterative multi-stage process designed to seek opinions and is recognised as useful in areas where there is little current research. Two rounds of the Delphi were completed and in the second round a consensus was reached on the skills and methods required for facilitation of work based IPL. The evidence that emerges from the data is described and discussed using examples from the panel and conclusions drawn. The chapter concludes with discussion on how this research was utilised within the other areas of the project and within the organisations involved.

The provision of high quality IPL in practice is essential as over the past decade, radical changes have occurred in the organisation and delivery of services across health and social care, with effective provision increasingly dependent on good team work and active cooperation across disciplines.[3,4] The move to a primary care led NHS in the UK,[5] the introduction of Children's Trusts, and the growing pressure for a service that is user-led has accelerated the demand for interprofessional and multi-agency education.[6,7] The value of IPL in the practice environment, Whittington and Bell[8] suggest, lies in the opportunities for professionals working alongside each other to learn together, creating a culture of collaboration. Anecdotal evidence from practice found that the majority of IPL in practice draws on traditional staff development models, delivered through short courses and workshops, or focused on post-registration continuing professional development.[9] Most professionals are juggling a high workload alongside their commitments to lead IPL sessions and whilst in practice there is little or no funding for IPL, there is also a range of potential interprofessional learning that presents opportunistically. The majority of IPL in practice occurs where service activities are based and usually addresses organisational need, often as quality improvement initiatives. However, much of the research highlights the failure of this learning to achieve improvements in collaborative working;[10] the tragic consequences of which are highlighted in many recent cases such as the Laming and Kennedy enquiries.[11,12]

An opportunity to explore the preparation of facilitators for work-based IPL and to provide some answers was the remit of one of the four schemes of the PIPE project. The particular challenge was to try and find out if there are additional skills and knowledge needed for facilitation of interprofessional learning in the workplace. Observation of interprofessional learning events in practice suggests that the facilitators involved with interprofessional groups in practice situations find the process difficult. Frequently in practice this remit falls to professionals such as GPs, doctors, nurses and allied health professionals in specialist areas, for example in areas such as palliative care, diabetic care or child protection. Although they may have a significant expertise in their chosen field, professionals facilitating IPL groups frequently say that they feel ill prepared for the role. Evidence for this is mostly anecdotal from practice but in the evaluation of a government funded initiative[13] it was identified that the outcome of the learning experience depended on the quality of facilitation skills which were often assumed, but not always present. The notion that an expert practitioner in the field of health and social care also has the skills to facilitate a group of professionals with the aim of promoting IPL can be a misguided assumption. Meanwhile, the dearth of research into the preparation of facilitators leaves largely unanswered the question whether the acquisition of additional facilitation skills would enhance the process of shared, work-based learning. In reality, with participant feedback regularly suggesting that poor facilitation affects the quality of the shared learning experience, these people appear insufficiently equipped for this challenging and demanding educational role. Certainly the widespread practice of appointing IPL facilitators on the basis of their expertise should be questioned as it does little for the confidence of the professionals involved as outlined in Box 3.1.

The premise at the beginning of the project was that there were recognisable transferable skills used by all facilitators working with different professions. These were described as fundamental skills and enhanced skills. Facilitation of IPL in the

BOX 3.1 Interprofessional learning in practice

In many areas there are now regular training programmes for basic awareness of child protection that are considered to be mandatory training for all employees within organisations, as an outcome of the Laming Enquiry.[11] The days are usually facilitated by a rotating group of professionals from different agencies on a voluntary basis. In this example the session was co-facilitated by a recently appointed specialist nurse for child protection and a representative from educational welfare. On this particular day it was a large group of people from many organisations. There were two participants who were annoyed they had to attend as they insisted they have little contact with children. They refused to engage in the groupwork and became quite argumentative in the feedback session. Both of the facilitators found the situation difficult to manage and were concerned at the impact the tension had had on the other learners. Following this incident one of the facilitators reported that she had lost her confidence and was reluctant to participate in further training sessions.

workplace, it was assumed, would require greater levels of skill to address issues of power, stereotypes, leadership and feelings of being de-valued in a multiprofessional setting. These areas are often not dealt with because of the inexperience of facilitators who may fear conflict and be unsure what the outcome will be if they challenge group members. The following framework was suggested as the basis of future model at the beginning of the project (Figure 3.1).

Brief outline of the PIPE three study

Following the outlining of the above framework and initial discussions, three questions emerged and continued to be asked throughout the work of the project:

- are the facilitation skills and knowledge necessary for facilitators of work-based interprofessional learning any different from the skills needed for facilitation of any other work-based group?
- if so, how should they be promoted?
- and crucially, how are they to be acquired?

This led to the following research question:

> What, if any, are the facilitation skills and knowledge needed to promote effective interprofessional learning in the workplace?

The research method utilised the Delphi technique which seeks to overcome some of the disadvantages found in the decision making process and, according to Crotty[14] is deemed an effective method for structuring group communication when dealing with a complex problem. The aim was to gather opinions and

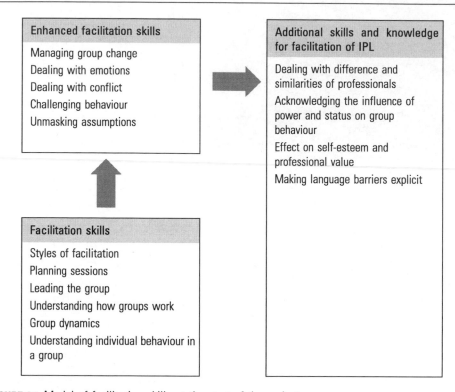

FIGURE 3.1 Model of facilitation skills at the start of the project.

inform the debate by ascertaining 'expert opinion' on the complexities of facilitating IPL.

Further information on the research process can be found in Appendix 2. The final outcomes of the process demonstrated that to prepare facilitators for IPL they need to acquire advanced and in depth skills of facilitation, similar to those required to facilitate other complex diverse groups. But more importantly the results produced some very rich data about the sort of skills, knowledge and teaching methods for IPL facilitation. The final results were then organised into five main themes (*see* Table 3.1) with these being the result of much discussion with the team and revisiting the data on a number of occasions. The findings will be used throughout this chapter and related to work-based learning in practice.

Findings from the study

Awareness and use of self as a facilitator

A recurring finding identified as essential to effective group facilitation was the ability and willingness to be reflective about the role.

Personal qualities and the effect of the facilitator's behaviour, demonstrated through their value and belief systems, were shown to play a key role in effective

TABLE 3.1 Five themes from Delphi data

1 Awareness and use of self as a facilitator.	Personal qualities: an awareness of ways own behaviour can influence group and outcomes. Potential role conflict: an awareness of own professional identity and personal bias, e.g. own identity is secondary to group needs. Confident risk taking: a willingness to tackle sensitive issues and to challenge stereotypical, racist, sexist or ageist statements. Reflective practice: making a conscious effort to monitor own performance in the process of facilitating. Objectivity: making statements in the light of available evidence whilst acknowledging differing view points. Open mindedness: not making assumptions about individuals and groups.
2 Dealing with difference and conflict.	Making time to explore differences and commonalities. Being aware of diversity. Challenging views expressed and not the person expressing them. Recognising that, although it may remain hidden, conflict is natural and can be creative. Avoiding the use of professional jargon.
3 Group process and relationships.	Being explicit on aims and desirable outcomes. Remaining flexible and helping the group make choices and decisions. Openly reviewing and revising outcomes. Actively facilitating the social dimensions of group learning about other professional roles. Recognising participants may have own agenda. Keeping scenarios, role play, etc work-based and authentic. Recognising the importance of evaluating the interprofessional dimension of group. Reflecting on and responding to feedback from group.
4 Power dimensions: facilitator and group.	Acknowledging organisational power and status, e.g. that many professionals work in hierarchical institutions. Understanding that power relations are linked with role stereotypes and professional groups. Being aware that an unequal power base affects individual perceptions, identities, behaviours and beliefs. Being aware of own power, i.e. that the facilitator does not remain 'neutral'. Empowering all in the group to participate.
5 Context and planning.	Facilitation skills are best developed when: ■ sessions are pre-planned ■ prior consideration is given to sensitive or contentious issues ■ practical matters and external factors that may impact on the session, e.g. organisational policies, processes, procedures, and, in some cases, politics, are taken into account ■ workplace culture ensures commitment and support at all levels.

IPL outcomes. Individual identity is so closely linked to self-image and self-esteem that the behaviour of the facilitator must influence and impact on the group. Consequently a facilitator may provide either a negative or positive response to an incident simply because his or her own emotional buttons have been pressed. Therefore, the ability to reflect on one's own role was seen as an essential skill and affirms the anecdotal evidence of the importance of being self-aware as identified in the JUMP Project.[13]

Further, the literature on group dynamics refers to the skill of the facilitator to remain 'substantively neutral', which as Schwarz suggests, is the ability to 'express no preference for any solutions the group considers'.[15] This notion of neutrality is reflected in a number of statements in the project feedback, for example:

> The ability to see both sides, to be personally uninvolved and objective, treat all individuals equally in all circumstances, not be drawn or manipulated into any position.

Helme and Sills[16] advise that to sustain IPL, teaching will be underpinned by a set of attitudes and behaviours of respect for other professions, trust and accountability, all of which require self-awareness and reflection. Recognition of these observations is implicit in many of the comments from the panel, but it remains unclear whether these qualities in themselves guarantee neutrality. Where an ability to be reflective and self aware may help facilitators find a degree of neutrality within this narrow role, it is difficult to see how they can filter out totally the many thoughts and feelings that must arise from all their personal and professional experiences. In this sense, the potential for role conflict is high and facilitators may be better prepared to deal with it if they recognise the likelihood. The following comments from panel members certainly support this suggestion:

> You need to be aware of your own history and expectations: you need to remain fascinated by what's actually happening, which you are inevitably a part of.

However, professional background can lend credibility as a facilitator, and many comments reflected the idea that IPL sessions should be designed and run by a small group representing the participants. This is supported by evidence from practice where those facilitating work based IPL are often specialists within the professional groups and have a responsibility as a role model for practice. It is clearly demonstrated that a significant aspect of interprofessional learning and teaching is respecting the views of others, and self awareness is required to achieve this, although bias as a facilitator is difficult to eradicate and needs to be acknowledged. On this basis, self awareness is vital in presenting a positive attitude, both verbally and non-verbally, and could be argued as an additional skill as an IPL facilitator.

IPL is according to Barr[17] grounded in adult learning theory with reflection as an approach to learning one of the key principles of adult learning theory.[18,19,20] Whilst the entire panel affirmed they had received training in adult learning processes, only 55% had a professional teaching qualification. Furthermore, only 15% of the panel would recommend a professional teaching qualification with the majority suggesting short courses and study days with the practitioner gaining experience through practice. Certainly, in practice it would be an unrealistic expectation for all facilitators of IPL to have a teaching qualification and it is the ability of the facilitator to help the individual reflect on their own learning and professional roles and focus on IPL issues in the group that was viewed as important. In addition, the ability of the facilitator to reflect-in-action to encourage a greater level of critical analysis and thus group learning, was viewed as a higher level skill. The increased reflective skills needed relate in part, to attitudes and behaviours, i.e. respect for others, responsiveness to difference and accountability in an organisation. The ability to become, not only reflective practitioners but also self-directed critical thinkers, is essential according to Parsell *et al*[21] to prepare good team members and communicators for collaborative working. This was clearly thought of as important by the panel:

> More in depth reflection for an IPL group ... and ... there is a need to reflect on what is being learned and how in an IPL group.

However, Moss[22] in relation to training social workers, refers to reflection as being 'one of the most labour intensive ways' of working and not an area for the unconfident and hesitant teacher, with the responsibility of the teacher being to ensure that learners are 'emotionally intact' at the end of each session. This certainly has implications for IPL and there were a number of comments echoing this and implying that reflection is more challenging for IPL, particularly in relation to dealing with conflict. The ability to remain objective, able to acknowledge one's bias, not to be drawn in and manipulated, being non-judgemental were all significant aspects of facilitator behaviour.

Dealing with difference and conflict

The issue of difference was raised in many ways and had a significant place in understanding IPL facilitation. This section produced evidence that seemed key to addressing teaching the different professional cultures and offers the potential for a deeper understanding of aspects of facilitation for IPL groups. In this category unsurprisingly, the IPL section contained far more information about exploring the nature of the different professions and stereotyping, than the section on general facilitation.

The importance of being aware of diversity within the group was highlighted, whilst the recommendation was to stress the importance of exploring the common denominator, not stereotyping and maintaining an interprofessional approach. All IPL groups must be given time and the opportunity to learn about other group members, exploring assumptions and myths about other professions. Reference is made to how irritating people find it when they realise assumptions are being made about them, for example, as if all nurses or doctors are the same race, age and gender. This links with the discussion on the Illeris[1] framework and the need to address the emotive element during IPL. The panel commented on the need to be confident to take risks and challenge the group over sensitive issues to re-establish group norms. For example, issues such as professional stereotypes, 'all nurses are bossy … all doctors never turn up'. This was first thought of as peculiar to IPL groups where general assumptions are often made about professional behaviours, which influence the way the group works and the outcomes. However, this is equally applicable to any diverse complex group when racist, ageist, and sexist statements are made and not addressed by the group. This reflects Robertson's[23] recognition of other important 'shapers' of group behaviour, such as those of race and gender where the individual becomes subordinate in IPL sessions, and is a product of the profession. Therefore, no acknowledgment is given to the diversity of the group and consequently issues relating to gender and culture are frequently not addressed by the facilitator. Valuing people as individuals, first and foremost rather than labelling and generalising about professions/cultures, etc is essential for effective facilitation, as any IPL group is first and foremost a diverse group of people. The importance of this was demonstrated in the following statements:

> I would see peoples' different professional roles as just one aspect of the diversity that there is in most groups – age, gender, race, experience, sexual orientation.

> A key learning point for some might be the existence of other world views, value systems, etc than their own.

Conflict was a continuing theme throughout and is seen as antagonism or tension between any of the group members or the facilitator. The consensus was that it is no more common in IPL sessions as all active learning groups will experience conflict which should be viewed as natural and to be used creatively. There is a need to challenge the view, not the person and to focus on the issue and not the personality, whilst confronting in a positive and constructive way. Another observation was that conflict can remain hidden, professionals are often on their best behaviour in the IPL arena or participants withdraw as they are reluctant to raise something they see as contentious for fear of causing trouble. Consequently, this 'unspoken' conflict is crucial as it would have a negative impact on group process and requires particular skill as a facilitator, to constructively identify and discuss contentious issues. The implications of this behaviour on collaborative working are considerable, with Freeman *et al*[24] implying it will ultimately affect how the learner interprets aspects of teamwork.

It was also suggested that 'sometimes members of IPL groups like to jeopardise the groups or "score points" off the facilitator' with this behaviour being more common than conflict in IPL groups. Undoubtedly, this is significant as much of work-based IPL opportunities revolve around statutory and mandatory training, where the participants have been told to attend by their directorate, so is relevant for those facilitating IPL in practice. Lizzio and Wilson refer to the participant's willingness to engage in the task as depending on the extent to which they consider they have a choice in attending.[25] However, their advice is that many of these beginning 'states' can be positively influenced, by using specific interventions to enhance people's sense of choice.

What emerges from this research is that conflict can take many different forms and that skills and methods to address conflict need to be developed by those facilitating in order to maximise the learning opportunity. The significance for IPL is that tension may remain hidden, with participants either withdrawing or causing disagreement which can manifest as 'point scoring' off the facilitator. Consequently, it is important that the facilitator has open-minded acceptance to differing viewpoints and value systems, ones that may well clash with that of the facilitator or the group's own. Acknowledging the existence of other world views, giving space to hear these views requires skilful management and balance by the facilitator but is a skill required for effective facilitation of any complex diverse group.

Group process and relationships

Establishing group trust, explicit aims on the purpose of the session and achieving credibility, as a facilitator were the central issues in this category. Valuing people as individuals and using their experience in the group are the basic principles of adult education and these qualities are emphasised throughout this section. The centrality of using experiences from the workplace and encouraging problem solving gained high consensus. Whilst the importance of process, planning and organisation alongside the use of reliable resources was seen as essential.

Running any IPL session should have a large degree of flexibility to help the group make choices, to allow individuals in the group to develop and to encourage flexible outcomes. Constantly reviewing and revising the programme with the group should enable this to happen and was considered part of the adaptable approach necessary to facilitate IPL groups. Whilst the replies to this category were complex, there were a number of themes that emerged emphasising this skill as a facilitator.

The first theme related to the purpose of the work-based IPL and the conflicting outcomes required from the group process. Comments related to the organisational outcomes and that:

> The learning is for service development, or ... develop group objectives in line with service requirements.

These comments reflect current practice identified in the literature review, that most work-based IPL is provided by employing organisations as a training event with a specific purpose: for example, child protection training. It raises the question of how facilitators can have flexible outcomes and allow individuality to maximise the IPL potential, when they are constrained by service requirements to provide a content learning outcome. The paradox is that most of the current work-based training is about giving information and gives little recognition to the group process necessary to support IPL or to develop collaborative working:

> Some people feel that courses are about giving information; I would argue that it is much more about the people who deliver it.

Facilitation of the social dimension of the group is fundamental to group dynamics but in time limited sessions this has to be done with care as when an interprofessional group meets there is often a period of uncertainty, either voiced or silent. Appropriate use of ice-breakers, sensitive to the diverse groups needs and to the level of disclosure that feels comfortable is important. Learning about each other's professional roles is part of this essential process and variety of ways were suggested of developing the group and facilitating the process. Difficulties may arise as often a group meets together for a short period of time in a training session, consequently they will need to work rapidly through the stages of the group process.

The other area that was highlighted within IPL is the importance of not using professional jargon as it blocks communication and causes confusion when working with other agencies.

Participants come to groups bringing a variety of issues with them, such as past experiences of IPL sessions, learning styles that can make groupwork uncomfortable, unrealistic expectations, various work issues and personal baggage. This hidden agenda impacts on the decision making process and a multi-dimensional group learning together will need to find ways to make democratic decisions. The facilitator has a key role in ensuring the quiet voices are heard and the process is seen by all to be democratic and fair.

Furthermore, evaluation of the collaborative dimension in the group is imperaive and it was suggested that it requires reflection and review of both the individual learning and IPL. Evaluation appeared to be mostly for the benefit of organisations sponsoring training with the consensus that it was difficult to evaluate the interprofessional outcomes. There was evidence to suggest that success in practice based IPL depends on institutional support, the status of participants, positive expectations, a cooperative atmosphere, as well as a concern for and understanding of differences in the group.[26]

To summarise, the findings in this category highlight the importance of the facilitators' role in paying attention to the group process and links back to the Illeris[1] framework with the need to address the societal elements during IPL training. Whilst the facilitator is not solely responsible for what the learners bring with them to the learning environment, creating an atmosphere that values the individual and each contribution, and encourages them to engage will maximise the interprofessional learning in the group.

Power dimensions for facilitator and group

The main points emerging from this theme made reference to the discussion of stereotypes within professional groups and awareness of potential conflict. However, it was interesting that in the section relating to general group facilitation, there were as many references to dealing with different attitudes and emotions, as within the IPL section. Nevertheless, there was also evidence of a specific recognition that if not handled carefully, this behaviour would impede progress and learning of the group. This brings us back again to the tensions identified by Illeris[1] in the previous chapter with the importance of understanding the psychodynamic process involved with motivation and emotions and the societal impact associated with communication and interaction with the outside organisations, agendas, etc.

Learning to be a professional involves a process of socialisation distinctive to each professional group and the unequal power base between professions has significant and far-reaching implications for understanding the process of collaborative work.[23] Power plays a significant role in IPL and it demands the skill of the facilitator to be aware of the differentials and work with the group to achieve a level of trust and to encourage all to contribute. This was reinforced frequently in evidence from the panel, with many recommendations of the necessity of exploring professional roles, establishing the nature of professional conflict in the group and discussing career and training differences. Ultimately, it was recognised that the transition between sensible exploration of shared knowledge and 'ownership' of the specialism carries the possibility of a degree of resistance to sociocultural change, as one of the panel states:

> It is easy to be too ambitious, as changes in professional attitudes do not happen overnight.

However, this demands a certain level of skill and raises the wider question of how to address power dynamics with Humphris and Hean[27] suggesting that the flexibility needed to deliver IPL, will be dependent on other professionals challenging the existing medical 'hegemony'. Nevertheless, power is about more than just the medical profession and is a force that affects the individual's perceptions, identities, behaviour and beliefs. Many of the professions within health and social care have hierarchical organisational structures within their own disciplines, as well as in relation to other professions. The findings support this but also recognise the importance of sometimes accepting there may be a power discrepancy:

> It is unrealistic (and not true) to expect a junior receptionist to believe she has equal power to a senior doctor who may also be her employer – but nevertheless she must see that she has much of value to offer.

The differential power bases of professional groups impacts on participants who do not feel competent to engage in the group activities. Skills are needed to enable the differences to be used constructively within the group as there is a danger the power differentials remain hidden during group activities, but continue to fuel conflict. This again emphasises the importance of recognising the value of the individual and not the professional. Furthermore, Gilmartin[28] points out that the shift from the expert status of a teacher to that of facilitator might also involve a perceived loss of power. The panel highlighted the self confidence and awareness necessary to acknowledge ones own limitations:

> I find it can be a strength to acknowledge your own limitations.

Finally, the evidence highlights the importance of the facilitator being aware of their own power as although it may offer credibility to the group, it also brings with it the associated differentials and professional stereotypes. Interprofessional learning brings with it many complexities and it is the combination of personal and professional qualities as a facilitator that enables the learner to maximise their opportunity to engage and learn from the group.

Context and planning

The evidence that emerged from the data suggested that skills and teaching for facilitation cannot be developed without addressing the context, planning and authenticity of the process in which IPL occurs.

Pre-planning the session: to establish in advance information about the participants, awareness of any contentious issues and agreement on the sponsor's aims and objectives for the session. There was a plethora of information on how to set up groups, the importance of ice-breakers, ground rules and the use of resources:

> Using a mixture of styles of activities to encourage everyone to participate.

> Whenever possible work on problems/scenarios which require collaborative teamwork.

Many of the panel recognised how important it was to ascertain from the organisers in advance, information about the participants, any controversial issues, and the organisation's aims and objectives of the session. Much of the information could have related to the setting up of any group and this was recognised by the panel. Practical issues of adaptable rooms with chairs that can be moved, the timing for the session, refreshments, resources and administration to all participants play a key role in successful IPL session.

The attitude and learning environment is strongly influenced by external factors such as the different health and social care organisations, policies that shape practice, other health and social care personnel, service users, professional beliefs, and career pathways. Although this agenda is unlikely to be explicit it is an extra dimension for the facilitator and adds to the complexity of the facilitation process for IPL. Furthermore, there is a responsibility on organisations sponsoring learning to be supportive of the ethos of IPL and clear about the purpose and outcomes of any initiatives. Finally, in addition, workplace culture needs commitment and support at all levels and the learning must relate to the work of the real day-to-day problems that practitioners face in the multi-agency, multiprofessional culture in which they practice.

Whilst the distinction needs to be drawn between an interprofessional learning opportunity in practice and shared learning for service requirements, strategies are necessary to maximise the opportunistic learning in practice to further collaborative working.[27] The indications are that the panel believe it is the process of effective group facilitation that enables the student to have a wider perspective of emerging culture and knowledge particularly relevant to IPL. They need to understand the learning process, by which the students will truly learn 'from and about each other' and provide appropriate training for those employees on whose shoulders this remit falls.

Implications and conclusion

This chapter discussed the research carried out by the PIPE scheme three project team and the implications of these findings for practice. The motivation to undertake this research emanated from the concerns in practice of the number of professionals facilitating work based IPL without preparation or training for the role. The questions that emerged were echoed throughout the work of the project, such as whether there are different facilitation skills and knowledge necessary for facilitators IPL and, if so, how can they be acquired? This research was well grounded in practice and there was consensus and agreement achieved in many areas whilst the process enabled identification of specific skills and knowledge that need to be acquired to facilitate IPL in practice. Although in many respects the findings showed the skills and teaching methods were similar for facilitation of IPL as for any other diverse group, what also became apparent was evidence from the panel that poor facilitation could inhibit the group process necessary to prepare practitioners for collaborative practice.

Further clarification is needed to distinguish the role of a trainer (or practice teacher) from that of facilitator. Although, in work-based IPL this is frequently a dual role, as group facilitator and trainer are likely to be the same person. Consequently, facilitators needs to be prepared for both roles, with a clear understanding of how group dynamics can impact on the learning environment but also how to maximise the interprofessional shared learning opportunities. Furthermore, there is a responsibility on organisations sponsoring learning, to be supportive of the ethos of IPL and clear about the purpose and outcomes of any initiatives. In the data there were many recommendations for practice that could be undertaken by facilitators as preparation for IPL. In addition, a multitude of factors emerged that could encourage or discourage IPL. Consequently, the research study did demonstrate that facilitators need to be prepared for IPL and should not be expected to lead groups without additional preparation.

In conclusion, the findings showed that experienced facilitators of IPL have the skills and teaching methods to promote effective work based IPL. However, it was also evident from the research findings that these skills and teaching methods were learnt over many years of experience, accompanied by some specific preparation as a facilitator. Following the completion of the Delphi, these findings were used within the other three PIPE schemes to investigate the implications for facilitators of IPL in the other areas of the project.

The next chapter reports on a research project carried out to explore the preparation of facilitators in the higher education institutions and the implications for postgraduate education programmes. The aim of the chapter is to make practical recommendations of ways in which IPL can be incorporated effectively into postgraduate learning and teaching programmes arising from the findings of PIPE scheme two.

CHAPTER 4

Embedding interprofessional learning in postgraduate programmes of learning and teaching

KATY NEWELL-JONES

Introduction

The challenge of how best to prepare health and social care professionals to promote effective interprofessional learning (IPL) has become an important question in curriculum development for postgraduate programmes in learning and teaching.

The aim of this chapter is make practical recommendations of ways in which IPL can be incorporated effectively into postgraduate learning and teaching programmes arising from the findings of PIPE scheme two. This will be achieved by exploring:

- the key challenges experienced by health and social care professionals in relation to their roles as lecturers, teachers and practice educators
- three types of learning experiences which participants on postgraduate education programmes felt promoted the development of interprofessional working practices
- the implications for curriculum development for MSc/MA education programmes.

PIPE scheme two involved educators from four higher education institutions (HEIs), each of which offered well-established MSc/MA education programmes. These programmes were very different in nature and attracted different cohorts of students from a wide range of nurses with a small number from other health professions to a generic MA education with a strong representation from health and social care but also including lecturers from other disciplines across the university. The historical commitment and driving forces relating to IPL were also different in each HEI. However, the overarching aim of the IPL component in all HEIs was to support the development of lecturers and practice educators to identify and use interprofessional opportunities for collaborative learning with the intention of positively promoting interprofessional working practices.

Brief outline of the PIPE two study

In January 2003, at the beginning of the PIPE project the broad research question for PIPE scheme two was, 'how can IPL most effectively be incorporated into teaching programmes?' Initial discussions explored both positive and interpretative research approaches.

The group agreed to a working research question which was:

> What are the key factors in promoting IPL in postgraduate programmes in teaching and learning?

Radnor's[1] framework for the analysis of qualitative interpretative data was used to analyse the data (*see* Figure 4.1). The research process using Radnor framework is to be found in Appendix 3. The findings from the research study will be used throughout this chapter and related to practice for curriculum developers and lecturers in higher education institutions.

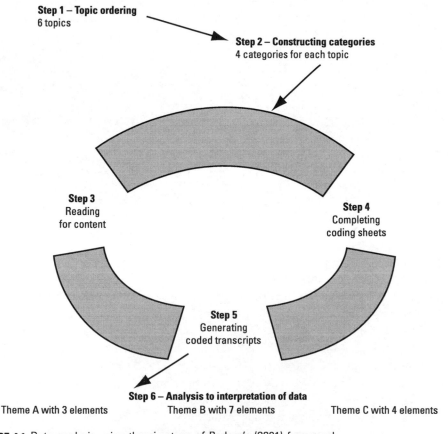

Step 1 – Topic ordering
6 topics

Step 2 – Constructing categories
4 categories for each topic

Step 3
Reading
for content

Step 4
Completing
coding sheets

Step 5
Generating
coded transcripts

Step 6 – Analysis to interpretation of data

Theme A with 3 elements   Theme B with 7 elements   Theme C with 4 elements

FIGURE 4.1 Data analysis using the six steps of Radnor's (2001) framework.

Findings from the study

The first stage of the analysis of the focus group's transcripts identified the key challenges of IPL, i.e. those factors which make interprofessional working more difficult in practice. These challenges are drawn from the experiences of more than 40 health and social care professionals who are actively engaged in postgraduate courses in learning and teaching whilst also working as educators in formal and non-formal contexts, in clinical and educational settings.

The second stage of the analysis identified which learning experiences were most influential in developing positive interprofesssional working practices. These are discussed in relation to curriculum development of postgraduate programmes in learning and teaching.

Key challenges in interprofessional learning

There was an overwhelming consensus on the key challenges identified by participants through the analysis of the transcripts from the focus groups. These were clustered under topics and categories following Radnor's framework (Table 4.1). There were no surprises in these challenges: the issues have all been identified

TABLE 4.1 Topics and categories identified from the focus groups (Radnor's framework)

Topics	Categories
Ambiguity of IPL	■ Perceptions and definitions ■ Motives for IPL ■ Barriers ■ When, who, with and how
Context, power and authority	■ Impact of IPL on individual's professional identity ■ Influence of policy, accreditation and resources on IPL ■ Professional differences and expectations ■ Power and status differences: profession, individual and institutional
Outcomes	■ Measurement of outcomes ■ Changes in working and thinking patterns to a more democratic environment ■ Improvement in patient/client care ■ Cost-cutting
Complexity of working and teaching interprofessionally	■ Levels of discourse ■ Challenges ■ Solutions
Role of the educator	■ Crossing professional boundaries ■ Modelling values of IPL ■ Skilled facilitation ■ Working positively with diversity of students/participants

and discussed in the literature on interprofessional learning. However, it was an important aspect of the study to draw out these issues in order to move on to considering how to address them most effectively when developing MSc/MA education programmes for health and social care professionals.

Ambiguity of IPL

Participants felt that the field of IPL was surrounded by ambiguities which were unsettling, confusing and sometimes overwhelming. Although they might have a clear idea about what they personally understood by IPL, participants had different definitions for the purpose of IPL in practice, some of which were in direct conflict with each other. For example, those who felt the primary purpose of IPL was cost-reduction and those who felt it was developing more effective working practices. The motives for, and barriers to, IPL differ radically in different contexts. Some HEIs were responding to the government's desire for IPL; others from a fundamental commitment to collaborative teamworking. Some clinical teams were responding to a belief that improved IPL could enhance patient care, whilst others were responding reluctantly to the pressures to include greater representation from across the professions in team meetings. Another unsettling feature was the logistics of delivering IPL with, for example, few clear-cut answers to whether IPL is most appropriate at pre- or post-registration.

There was a strong feeling that this ambiguity, in itself, was demoralising and led to many feeling it was extremely difficult to promote IPL with so little overall consensus on the purpose, definition and motives for IPL.

Context, power and authority

Context appears to be one of the most significant factors in IPL, with each situation having unique features suggesting that models and solutions also need to be uniquely tailored to each circumstance. Issues of power, hierarchy and authority dominate the discussion with language of war and conflict often being used. Individuals talk of warring factions, competing agendas, of groups dominating or suppressing others and of lacking authority or being overpowered or disempowered. The impression given was largely that people felt that they were powerless to change the status quo and that power was often used inappropriately.

Outcomes

There was considerable confusion about the intended outcomes of IPL with many feeling that the key motive was to cut costs. People were unclear about the intended outcomes, although many had a personal commitment to IPL as a means of enhancing interprofessional team working in practice and improving patient care. The difficulties in measuring outcomes of IPL were widely recognised.

Complexity of working and teaching interprofessionally

There was a strong recognition of the complexity of interprofessional working and teaching. This was reflected at the levels of individuals, teams, departments and institutions. Challenges were complex, with competing agendas and solutions were rarely straightforward.

Role of the educator

The role of the educator in interprofessional learning was seen as paramount. This requires skilled facilitation, the ability to work across professional boundaries, and to draw on the diversity and experience within the group.

Learning experiences which promote the development of interprofessional working practices

Having identified the key challenges to IPL experienced by participants the study moved on to identify the learning experiences which, in the opinions of the participants on postgraduate learning and teaching programmes, enable health and social care professionals to develop positive approaches to interprofessional working in the workplace – the ultimate aim of IPL. Three broad, interlinked themes were identified, each of which have a number of categories (Table 4.2).

TABLE 4.2 Topics and categories identified from the focus groups

Themes	Categories
A. Experiencing IPL as an approach to professional practice	■ Perceiving IPL as a way of relating to colleagues, rather than a set of teaching tools and techniques ■ Creating a climate conducive to IPL ■ Extending the value base of relating to other professionals with respect and valuing their role and perspective, to all professional relationships, educational and practice
B. Experiencing modelling of IPL in a variety of contexts, both educational and practice-based	■ The value of time invested at the beginning of any IPL initiative to enable the group to begin to see members as individuals ■ A commitment to collaborative learning by the facilitator ■ A mutual understanding that the process of learning is at least as important as the content ■ A fundamental belief that the learners are the most important learning resource present ■ The facilitator has the awareness, skills and willingness to deal with discrimination and conflict in positive ways which enable all present to learn from the process ■ The nature of the facilitator role is made very clear and will actively move between providing input to the group, facilitating the process and being a fellow learner ■ There is an understanding that the facilitator will invest part of themselves in the process
C. Opportunities to reflect on the challenges of IPL	■ The role of the educator in IPL contexts ■ Perceived, intended and expected outcomes of IPL ■ Barriers to IPL ■ Issues relating to power and hierarchy in IPL contexts

Theme A. Experiencing IPL as an approach to professional practice

The most important factor was viewing IPL as an approach to professional practice, rather than a skill set. Many first approached IPL assuming that they need to 'learn to do it effectively'. However, having studied IPL, they felt strongly that IPL was about developing a positive approach to talking about, and working with, other professionals when they were present and when they were not! Participants kept returning to the importance of the value base of IPL, for example:

> I think one of the interesting things about what you said is the value statement … it does have to be a philosophy, a value of the team and if it isn't then it doesn't work.

> Yes, a philosophy for the programme rather than for specific modules.

There are three interlinked components to this theme. Firstly that IPL is more concerned with attitude and approach, associated with valuing diversity in complex teams, than a set of tools and techniques to be 'adopted' in multiprofessional groups:

> You know an IPL teaching approach is about being aware of where people are coming from and how they perceive themselves and what their circumstances are.

Secondly, the importance of creating a climate within which interprofessional interactions are positive:

> It really makes you think what it means to be a health and social care educator in the widest sense, that you have to really step outside of your own professional box and re-think what you know as a profession-specific educator and what does that really mean in a wider context.

> I would go back to facilitating diverse complex groups, letting your own tendency to campaign on behalf of your own strong passions slip into the background and letting the facilitation of the learning process be paramount.

This aspect is explored further under the second theme of the modelling of IPL, where some of the aspects of creating a climate conducive to effective IPL are identified.

Thirdly, the need for the value base of IPL to be extended into all professional relationships of a lecturer or practice educator and not only evident in their educational role:

> To learn about other people's professions and respect other people's professions. And have more understanding of how people inter-relate and how people can, in the future, work across the professions and work together.

The key message from theme A, therefore, is the importance of participants being actively encouraged to think of IPL not in terms of a set of teaching tools and techniques, but in terms of establishing authentic and mutually respectful relationships. Health and social care professionals are acutely sensitive to the degree of competition, mutual respect and collaboration between professional groups. The outcomes are likely to be less successful when educators attempt to teach 'skills to manipulate members of different professional groups into behaving in different ways' rather than encouraging mutual understanding and assertiveness by all professional groups. Equally, educators who purport to support IPL, but in practice show less respect for groups not present are likely to encourage similar practices among participants. This is not to say that political correctness needs to dominate; some stereotyping is useful. Professional groups do differ and difference can be recognised, even humorously, but with respect!

Theme B. Experiencing modelling of IPL in a variety of contexts, both educational and practice-based

Theme B emphasises the value of students experiencing substantial modelling of effective IPL in both formal, educational and practice settings. By this I mean students actively participating in events involving a range of different professional health and social care groups. Where individuals actually experience effective IPL in different contexts, including classroom, practice settings, and institutional meetings, this appears to motivate them to incorporate IPL into their own practice to a greater extent:

> It's clearly evident that some students do see really, really good examples of interprofessional working and others don't and that seems to really motivate them...

The role of the facilitator in IPL was considered crucial and the focus groups identified the following characteristics which they felt were essential:

- the value of time invested at the beginning of any IPL initiative to enable the group, however large or small, to gain an overview of the make up of the group and begin to see members as individuals. The amount of time required for this aspect should not be underestimated
- a genuine commitment to collaborative learning on the part of the facilitator
- a mutual understanding that the *process of learning* is at least as important as the content and that this aspect therefore needs particular preparation time on the part of the facilitator
- a strong commitment that the learners are one of the most important learning resources present, in terms of learning with, from and about each other's roles and developing effective working practices. The preparation, therefore, needs to include activities designed to enable learners to learn from each other and not to assume that this will take place 'naturally' as part of the group process
- the facilitator has the awareness, skills and willingness to deal with discrimination and conflict in positive ways which enable all present to learn from the process. An important aspect of this is that the facilitator does not shy away from conflict him/herself, attempting to maintain a comfortable atmosphere at

all costs, but is able and willing to encourage groups to explore different perspectives

■ the nature of the facilitator role is made very clear and will actively move between providing input to the group, facilitating the process and being a fellow learner

■ there is an understanding that the facilitator will invest part of themselves in the process.

Theme B, therefore, emphasises the need for participants on postgraduate programmes on learning and teaching to experience as wide a range of 'IPL encounters' as possible. This theme links directly to theme C.

Theme C. Opportunities to reflect on the challenges of IPL

Theme C identified the value of providing students with specific opportunities to reflect on the challenges of IPL for themselves. It is not sufficient to be exposed to a range of IPL events. There was also a need for practical, regular activities, for example action learning circles or discussion groups where participants gained from structured reflection, made sense of their experiences and developed strategies for facilitating IPL effectively. There were four categories relating to this theme which participants emphasised.

Firstly, the role of themselves as educators in a variety of IPL contexts. Students came from diverse professional practices and valued time to discuss how the key elements of IPL identified above related to their own context and from this draw their own personal conclusions:

> … the danger that there are people doing it who are not really wanting to do it, doing it because they've got to. I've seen this in my placement area … people basically told to go and facilitate interprofessional learning who were just not interested. Some of them didn't even turn up. A lot of them weren't all that bothered about people working in an interprofessional way.

> … but if there isn't a chance in the actual session, you know, some people might go away and not really have found out about other roles.

Secondly, there was a wide range of perceived, intended and expected outcomes of IPL, some of which appeared to be motivational and others which might inhibit effective IPL. Participants appeared energised with regard to IPL when discussing perceived outcomes relating to improving patients' care and also to improved teamworking:

> … their own agenda; social workers, doctors, nurses. So when they are in a meeting with a patient they are looking after their own priorities, they don't know what the others are doing. So learning about each other would be very good and would be effective for patients in the long run.

> And I think have been quite a lot of … public examples in the media where that inter-connection has fallen down and not been working. I think one way

they can try to address that is to ... through interprofessional education. Bringing these people together.

Whereas when perceived outcomes include the development of a generic health worker, merging roles or saving money, participants were predictably less positive about IPL:

> ... some of the push for this is the changing roles of nurses and stuff which is driven by government saying 'Hey can we get nurses to do the stuff doctors did?'

Thirdly, a number of barriers to IPL were identified, many of which are surmountable given awareness and appropriate opportunities to discuss possible strategies to alleviate the problem, to reduce the tension or simply to make the most appropriate choice under the circumstances. The list of potential barriers raised by participants was extensive; the most frequently mentioned are discussed here. One of the most commonly raised barriers was the tension between covering the required content allocated to a session and allowing time for collaborative, interactive learning:

> ... it boils down to what content you have to cover – there isn't always time for the actual process of learning to evolve really is there?

Language continues to be raised as a barrier. Sometimes, the issue is the inadvertent use of acronyms or terms with which another professional group is unfamiliar:

> I find that when I go to the GP group that I belong to they have such an enormous amount of acronyms and things that I can't follow. They agree, I agree they don't understand the things that I can understand.

On other occasions it is not the use of technical jargon which causes tensions but the attitude between professional groups:

> I was quite shocked at how much interprofessional tension there is, so whatever group you're looking at in nursing, ODP, physio, or OTs ... And then you start discovering there are tremendous tensions between the different types of physios. There's tension between the physios and osteos – the osteopaths. There are tremendous tensions with the OTs. There are tremendous tensions within radiography and radiotherapy and so it goes on. ... between learning disability nursing and adult nursing and paediatric and, it's incredible how much tension there is within the professions.

Another barrier which is less well documented is the fear of interprofessional teaching being less valued than uniprofessional teaching as identified in the following statement:

> I do sometimes wonder, just sort of being quite a new lecturer, I have the slight impression that amongst some teams, teaching on interprofessional learning modules is seen to be a bit less high status thing to do than teaching on the specialist uniprofessional modules. ... and personally I think it is really important,

> IPL teaching takes a lot of skill but I know there are some people who think that it doesn't involve much preparation and it's an easy thing to do.

As IPL has succeeded in drawing together health and social care professional from a range of professional backgrounds so the pressure has increased to gain representation from all relevant professional groups. It was apparent that, at times, an enormous amount of effort has been directed towards achieving this goal. In the following example the names of the professional groups have been replaced with A, X, Y, and Z:

> It is getting everybody on board and I think most professionals want to go but the difficulty is that the Xs, they are the key. My example is child protection. When we used to do child protection training in the Trust everybody would come because they would see it as utmost importance but yet the As didn't and when it came to a case they didn't know what to do. And they would ask the Ys or the Z who was around if they went to the training and they did know what to do.

Finally, the findings in relation to power and hierarchy indicated two potentially contradictory findings. Hierarchical structures within and between the National Health Service and Social Care Service, and hierarchies within the higher education sector, are perceived as barriers to interprofessional learning and working. This is especially the case with the hegemony of the Russell Group of universities, (the nineteen most research-intensive universities in the UK), where the majority of medicine and dentistry education takes place. For example:

> As long as doctors are predominantly educated in these – so-called – elite establishments and nurses, midwives and health visitors in places such as this, there are going to be enormous difficulties unless we sort of break down barriers in the workplace and foster genuine interprofessional education.

However, the findings also indicated at the level of the group and the individual, that where IPL provided specific opportunities for students to explore issues relating to power and hierarchy in IPL, this often resulted in the development of more assertive practices in a wide range of group settings:

> I think it also helps people to explore, I think, some of the difficult issues about working in teams, which is about things like power and hierarchy ... the links with people in multiprofessional teams and so many of the big challenges when people come to be educators in the workplace are about these, especially if they are nurses, about their role in the team and how they might get undermined either by power and hierarchy and other people's perceptions or their own perceptions of their power.

Two examples were presented, the first where an experienced nurse felt the need to challenge the assessment practice of a multiprofessional team of which he was a member. Following an opportunity to explore the interprofessional relationships in the group, a fellow student reported:

.... he found that incredibly useful in that it had separated out for him what were issues of power and hierarchy, what were the issues of education ... where he was doing it [challenging] on a good education basis and where he was doing it in a poor, poor basis because he had not really explored the issues of power and hierarchy in the team.

The second example relates to a diabetes facilitator, working with a multiprofessional team:

... by the time she had finished looking at what her role was, what the power was and how her leadership style could be enhanced in terms of facilitating the group, she took a more pro-active role in that group. Interestingly the medics stood aside and let her do that and she was able to take her agenda forward.

In these examples, students had been provided with experiential opportunities for participants to explore issues of power and hierarchy in groups drawn from their profession, supported by the theory and practice of facilitating complex diverse groups.

Theme C, therefore, recognises that there are no simple set answers to the challenges which IPL poses but emphasises the value of providing opportunities for structured and supportive reflection. Participants on MSc/MA education programmes found bringing the issues which they encounter in practice to a safe environment to explore was effective in developing their confidence and skills in IPL:

... so that would be an important dimension in IPL ... engaging with groups you're not familiar with and building up your confidence in being able to interact with them.

Implications for curriculum development

Having considered the three types of learning experiences which appear to promote positive IPL working practices, these are now related to curriculum development in MSc/MA education programmes.

Perhaps surprisingly, the specific means by which IPL was incorporated into the MSc/MA programmes, whether by discrete modules or embedded into core attributes, was less important than the overarching approach to IPL experienced by the students on the programmes.

This study provides three themes for how the essential characteristics for IPL facilitation might be developed among healthcare professional involved either as students, or as programme team members, of MSc/MA education programmes for health and social care professionals. These themes shown in Table 4.2 are:

- theme A: experiencing IPL as an approach to professional practice
- theme B: experiencing modelling of IPL in a variety of contexts, both educational and practice based
- theme C: opportunities to reflect on the challenges of IPL including:
  - the role of the educator

– perceived and intended outcomes
– barriers and challenges to IPL
– issues of power and hierarchy in IPL contexts.

These elements do not themselves provide solutions to the complexity and challenges of IPL, but provide a secure framework within which those developing their skills as educators can develop their understanding of IPL and begin the process of making informed choices. They rely on problem solving and other active learning approaches, particularly in groups, which enable individual educators to resolve the challenges they face through dialogue and reflection.

There is a strong agreement between the findings from this study with those from PIPE scheme three which used a Delphi process to engage with expert IPL facilitators to explore the characteristics of the effective IPL facilitator. The Delphi study identified the following five themes:

1 awareness and use of self as a facilitator
2 dealing with difference and conflict
3 group process and relationships
4 power dimensions for facilitator and group
5 context and planning.

Although many of the expert panel in the Delphi study did not identify staff development initiatives as key factors in their own development as facilitators of IPL, it is interesting to note that in this study students recognised that they were developing the characteristics recognised by the panel as valuable through their MSc/MA programmes.

Theme A suggests that IPL should be presented on MSc/MA education programmes as a way of interacting as a professional and not as a set of teaching tools and techniques to be 'brought out' when facilitating multiprofessional groups. There are similarities here with anti-racist teaching or disability awareness programmes, where participants are encouraged to address their prejudices and to ensure that they are respectful towards those from other races or those who are disabled, whether or not they are present. This theme has clear implications for professional development among programme teams, where IPL is perceived by some members as a current trend, or a specific skill set to be acquired, as opposed to an approach to professional practice. In these instances there is a danger of IPE reinforcing existing stereotypes.[2] Programme teams might find that instead of asking 'who can teach IPE?', they would be better placed asking 'to what extent do we as a team model effective IPL?' and 'how do we relate to each other across our professional boundaries?' In many teams there is further work needed in this area, raising awareness of the ways in which professional groups talk about each other, sometimes unaware of the subtle implications behind their language. Programme teams could, for example, invite the participants to feedback on the ways in which members of the programme team talk about other professional groups during teaching sessions and the extent to which team members use examples from professional contexts other than their own. Programme teams can also allocate specific time at the end of curriculum planning sessions to discuss the interprofessional relationships in the team. Sometimes an outside observer is valuable to draw attention to patterns which might be hidden from the team.

Themes B and C are closely linked. Theme B suggests that curriculum development should include identifying a range of opportunities for participants to experience modelling of IPL, i.e. having opportunities to experience and analyse events involving different professional groups. If the student cohort includes a number of professions there will be opportunities for modelling IPL within the course contact time. If the cohort is uniprofessional, or includes only a limited number of professional groups, then opportunities need to be designed into the programme. However, additional opportunities also need to be identified outside the formal teaching time, in practice settings and placements.

However, participating in, or observing, IPL events is not enough to develop the skills for effective facilitation of IPL! Health and social care professionals also need to dedicate time to discuss their role, their fears, hopes and challenges around interprofessional working and practice. They valued structured opportunities to discuss what went on, how different people responded, the balance of participation between professional groups, any power dynamics, the processes of decision-making, and most importantly, the role of the facilitator(s) and their interventions. It was essential that these reflections took place in a safe space where they could be honest about their feelings and issues, not a space where political correctness might stifle honest communication and debate.

Although clearly it is valuable to observe and participate in IPL which is effective, participants also learnt considerably from IPL which was problematic. Through analysing situations where there was excessive tension or conflict, or where one professional group did not participate or felt marginalised, participants developed alternative strategies for dealing with similar situations. For example, where the learning outcomes obviously related primarily to one professional group, other professional groups were likely to find the session less positive and on occasions could be detached or disruptive.

Some of the most successful learning experiences on the postgraduate programmes on learning and teaching, in terms of developing skills for dealing with difficult interprofessional situations, came from a specific module on facilitating complex diverse groups. This module used experiential learning and encouraged participants to discuss power, hierarchy and competing agendas in groups and to explore their own role in establishing and maintaining power differentials in multiprofessional groups. Other valuable learning opportunities included action learning circles with a focus on analysing interprofesional interactions. There were examples where those who felt disempowered in multiprofessional groups were encouraged to be more assertive and take responsibility for playing a stronger role, rather than assuming that others wanted them to play a submissive role and being angry at this situation. Exploring the emotional aspects of IPL often led to recognition of the role of emotion in inhibiting the rational analysis of interprofessional interactions. Once this was recognised, the educator could usually adopt a more detached approach and facilitate more effectively. The insights and skills developed through these discussions were applicable to other contexts involving complex diverse groups.

Although interprofessional education tends to focus primarily on multiprofessional programmes, the author suggests that these three themes are equally applicable to uniprofessional teacher preparation programmes. PIPE scheme one focused on increasing the interprofessional nature of the postgraduate diploma in Medical Teaching offered by the Oxford Deanery and validated through Oxford Brookes University. The student cohort continues to consist almost entirely of general practitioners (GPs), which has advantages in terms of meeting the specific needs of this professional group. However, substantial progress has been made in the way in which GPs engage with other professionals in their practice and use them in supporting the education of GP registrars, through changing the nature of the tutor team from uniprofessional to interprofessional. This has resulted in the values of IPL being incorporated into the core elements of the postgraduate programme and reflected in the assessment tasks. This process might not go as far as would be the case if the cohort became interprofessional, but through embedding the principles of IPL, modelling it and providing opportunities for the challenges to be aired and discussed, GPs were able to adopt more interprofessional ways of working as trainers in their practices.

In conclusion, PIPE scheme two has identified three priorities for consideration in developing postgraduate programmes in teaching and learning. These will support the development of lecturers and practice educators able and willing to identify and use interprofessional opportunities for collaborative learning with the intention of positively promoting interprofessional working practices.

CHAPTER 5

Preparing facilitators for interprofessional learning

BEE WEE AND JAN GOLDSMITH

Introduction

In earlier chapters of this book, it has been emphasised that there is a necessity to recognise that facilitators of interprofessional learning (IPL) do not need a unique set of skills, but that they need to develop the more advanced type of skills that would be required to facilitate any complex, diverse group. This implies that facilitators cannot simply be thrown in the deep end, even if they are used to managing homogenous groups effectively.

The aims of this chapter are to:

- discuss the premise of facilitation as a professional practice in education
- propose recommendations for the way in which facilitator preparation for IPL could effectively take place, taking into account the findings from the PIPE project.

The role of facilitating IPL requires specific preparation. The evidence for this statement comes from the findings of the research undertaken within PIPE schemes two and three, and evidence which arose from the work in PIPE schemes one and four as well as from a growing body of literature.[1,2,3,4] The findings from PIPE scheme three indicate that, currently, facilitators do not feel that they have been offered sufficient preparation before undertaking IPL within the workplace. It is not within the scope of this chapter to explore the reasons for such failure to adequately prepare facilitators, though one explanation might be a genuine but simplistic lack of appreciation that IPL groups are inherently complex and diverse, not just made up of several homogenous groups of individuals coming together.

Facilitation as a professional practice

Facilitators of learning are engaged in educational practice. Aristotle, as cited by Carr[5] suggests that in educational practice, the professional is frequently faced with competing choices and has to exercise practical wisdom, a combination of good judgement and action, knowing what is required in a particular moral situation and being willing to act on this knowledge. Hogan describes a facilitator as 'process consultant', who makes considered and deliberate interventions into how a group is working, helps group members become more aware of their functioning or enables them to achieve tasks that they could not have completed alone.[6] Because IPL settings are inherently complex and diverse situations, IPL facilitators need to constantly demonstrate professional artistry, described by Schon as the kinds of competence that practitioners display in 'unique, uncertain and conflicted situations of practice'.[7]

The authors' premise is that IPL facilitators engage in educational practice as professionals and are called upon to act with practical wisdom in uncertain situations. Insight into their own professional practice is a fundamental aspect of facilitator preparation. Such insights are developed not just through the acquisition of theoretical knowledge but through the range of experiences that each individual has undergone. Consideration of ways in which these two aspects can be combined to ensure the optimum outcome in a given situation is the essence of reflective practice.[8] However, as alluded to by Schon,[7] this process can be seen as an art or a skill in itself and as such, is something which needs to be worked on and developed over time through a structured approach. Indeed, it has been suggested that expertise in reflective practice can be seen to develop through a series of stages.[9]

Fish and Coles[10] offers the iceberg as a useful metaphor for professional practice. They invited a number of experienced healthcare professionals to reflect upon an incident they each took from their practice, write individually about this and then engage in critical discussion about their reflections as a group. Several aspects of their findings have particular relevance for facilitator preparation in IPL:

■ the realisation, by these professionals, that their professional actions (decisions and judgements) were determined more by their own values, beliefs and assumptions than by formal theories that they had encountered

■ the recognition that the learning had to be experienced and could not simply be passed on by others who had gone through a similar experience; greater understanding of their practice came through experience, personal reflection and deliberation with others.

Through this work and their deliberations with the group of participants, Fish and Coles[10] suggested that the iceberg would be a useful metaphor for professional practice, parts of it protruding above the waterline and visible, other parts not easily seen (Figure 5.1).

The aspects of professional practice, whether in healthcare, teaching or facilitating, which are part of the iceberg seen above the waterline are those actions which are visible. This might be evident in the behaviour which facilitators exhibit in response to conflict situations within IPL workshops, for example, irritation, avoidance or confrontation. The factors which influence facilitators' behaviours in response to such situations are often not visible, even to the facilitators themselves. These may include their previous experiences of similar situation, their expecta-

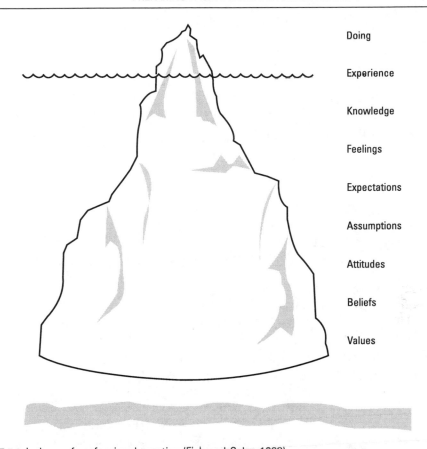

Doing

Experience

Knowledge

Feelings

Expectations

Assumptions

Attitudes

Beliefs

Values

FIGURE 5.1 Iceberg of professional practice (Fish and Coles 1998).

tions and assumptions about the participants and their beliefs and values. The opportunity to expose and reflect on the aspects of professional practice beneath the 'waterline' provides the facilitator with the opportunity to learn from that experience and develop his/her skills at a deeper level. An example is shown in Box 5.1 to illustrate this.

The findings from the PIPE project support this need to develop aspects of practice that are less visible, i.e. it is not so much the development of skills for doing what needs to be done (more technical skills) as much as how it needs to be done (process skills and skills to respond to situations). There needs to be opportunity for facilitators to reflect upon, and learn from, the process of IPL facilitation within a safe setting. The iceberg metaphor offers a structured approach to reflection in a step-by-step way.

Dimensions of learning

Earlier in this book, others have referred to the three dimensional model of learning described by Illeris.[11] Not only do facilitators need to develop insight into the

BOX 5.1 Facilitating IPL: application of iceberg model

Context:

IPL workshop consisting of two students from each of the following backgrounds: medical, nursing, occupational therapy, physiotherapy, social work: one facilitator.

Scenario:

The medical and nursing students begin to get into a heated discussion about their respective roles on a ward. Medical students stated that they felt unwelcome and were made to feel 'in the way'. The nursing students stated that they could see why the medical students felt that way because, unlike the nursing students who participated in patient care, medical students appeared to only follow their seniors around. They suggested that medical students might feel better if they started making a real contribution to patient care too.

Facilitator response:

Agreed with the nursing students about their perception and asked medical students how they could change their behaviour so that they would be perceived more positively on the ward. This was the 'doing' that was the only bit visible to all the workshop participants. The facilitator became obviously irritated with the medical students when they could not come up with a list of action points and, instead, wanted to explore further why they were made to feel 'in the way'. By the end of the workshop, the medical students left feeling resentful and that this workshop had been a waste of time; the nursing students left feeling that the medical students had been negative; the facilitator left feeling that the medical students had been 'difficult' and had made this a difficult event to facilitate.

What was really going on beneath the iceberg:

The facilitator came from a ward nursing background, so the nursing students' observation resonated with previous real life experience. The facilitator was also experienced in working with junior doctors in the clinical setting, with whom robust discussions about the role of medical students on the ward had taken place. This had not been particularly negative, so the facilitator's assumption was that such a discussion could usefully take place in this IPL workshop setting with the medical students. However, the facilitator had not taken into account the very different setting in which this discussion was taking place, the power relationship the facilitator had over these students (unlike the much more equal relationship possible in the clinical setting) and the fact that such a diverse group meant that the medical students might feel unsafe and picked on. Moreover, the facilitator's own values included a strong conviction that medical students' learning usually got in the way of patient care and smooth operation of the clinical service. In this situation, the facilitator failed to recognise this deep underlying value and to hold it safely in order to be able to facilitate and support all the students (medical, nursing and others) involved in this situation in an equitable manner.

hidden depths of their own professional practice, they also need to be able to hold the tension between the cognitive and emotional dimensions of learning, and between the learning process that takes place at an individual level and at the level of interaction with others. This is not always easy or predictable even in uniprofessional groups. When two or more professions come together to learn with, from and about each other in order to improve collaboration and the quality of care, the need to balance the cognitive, emotional and societal dimensions of learning, and to pay attention to both content and process, is even more crucial, but can result in much richer learning. This was a process that became evident in scheme four which functioned as a learning set. The documented reflections of the scheme four members, at the end of each meeting, demonstrate the richness of this learning with, from and about each other.

Illeris' framework[11] may be used by IPL facilitators to identify where their initial focus lies and to map out the process of the IPL event, in terms of where it sits in the framework at any one time. This framework provides a useful tool, both in preparing for an event and reflecting on it afterwards, to pay mindful attention and make careful choices about balancing the content and process of the IPL experience.

In the next part of this chapter, we draw together the findings from all of the schemes within the PIPE project and discuss these in terms of the implications for facilitator preparation. The discussion focuses around six themes which are:

1   development of self awareness
2   respecting and valuing difference
3   the impact of group dynamics on learning
4   managing issues around power and hierarchy
5   planning IPL
6   the facilitator's learning philosophy.

Emerging themes from PIPE project: implications for facilitator preparation

Development of self awareness

The expert panel in scheme three Delphi study were unanimous in their view that self awareness, acknowledgement of personal biases and awareness of own professional identity were essential qualities for IPL facilitators. Whilst such biases were inevitable (perhaps even adding to the richness of learning), it was seen as essential that facilitators were able to identify and acknowledge these within their teaching. This also emerged as a fundamental quality for IPL facilitators within scheme two, as facilitators' ability to use themselves as a 'tool' for learning was seen as important, as was their ability to act as an equal participant within the group, role modelling the importance of acknowledging personal beliefs and biases. In essence, if facilitators can acknowledge their own biases and values with the group and demonstrate how they deal with them (role modelling), then there is a good chance that the group will begin to do the same. Self awareness has been described as an essential attribute for reflective practitioners.[7] This quality, however, relies on individuals being aware of their own values, beliefs and prejudices in the first place, i.e. being able to dip beneath the water level and see the more hidden aspects of professional practice, as in the iceberg model (*see* Figure 5.1). Scheme four provided opportunity for such acknowledgement to take place within the safe setting of the learner set.

The development of a high level of self awareness and self knowledge therefore appears to be fundamental to professional practice, particularly so in the arena of facilitating interprofessional learning. It is essential that IPL facilitators are given regular opportunities to reflect upon and analyse their teaching practice in a similar way that clinicians are encouraged to do in clinical practice. These sessions could, therefore occur in a similar way to that of clinical supervision, i.e. they could occur in a group, or on a one-to-one basis. However, as with clinical supervision, a very important factor would be that an appropriate person takes the role of facilitator.[12] This person would themselves need to be a self aware, experienced IPL facilitator who could provide the degree of challenge necessary to enable individuals working at this level to explore alternative approaches to practice and to grow and develop both personally and professionally. The importance of being able to challenge traditional models and approaches to practice was demonstrated clearly within scheme one. For people in dual teaching and clinical roles, just as much emphasis should be given to developing the teaching element of their role as the clinical elements. The iceberg metaphor may be used to provide a safe and structured opportunity, through individual reflection and group deliberation, for IPL facilitators to develop their self awareness within sessions for facilitator preparation or reflection on real experiences.

Respecting and valuing difference

Understanding the variety of issues relating to diversity and difference within groups is another important issue for IPL facilitators. In scheme three, aspects such as awareness of the range of factors which make some groups more diverse than others, the importance of taking time to explore the differences and commonalities within groups and the difficulties associated with the use of professional jargon were highlighted. The findings indicate that facilitators need to be willing and able to challenge group members but that it should be the view that is challenged, not the person expressing that view. The panel also considered that conflict within any group is inevitable but, well facilitated, this may be harnessed as a positive and creative force. However, managing conflict appropriately is arguably a skill which particularly needs to be developed by IPL facilitators, as conflict is more likely to arise in complex, diverse groups and, managed inappropriately or left to fester, becomes destructive. Findings from scheme two suggested it was crucial for facilitators to be active in promoting non-discriminatory practice and to role model this throughout group sessions. The learner sets in PIPE scheme four provided opportunity to practice the skill of unpicking and valuing differences and the assumptions that underpin these. The example in Box 5.1 demonstrates how the facilitator's failure to recognise the diversity within the group meant that the medical students within that group were challenged in a somewhat unsafe context.

Awareness of the nature of, and issues surrounding, discriminatory practice would therefore appear to be essential, particularly when such practice lies deep beneath the surface. Here again, the use of the iceberg metaphor may provide a structured way for facilitators to explore their own values and beliefs which underpin their practice.

The impact of group dynamics on learning

The ability to be able to manage group dynamics to enable group members to develop effective working relationships was a key theme which emerged from PIPE schemes two, three and four. Facilitators were required to remain flexible within IPL sessions, allowing groups to develop their own identities. The ability to be able to actively facilitate the social dimension of the group, allowing individuals to get to know one another and subsequently learn about each other's professional roles, was seen as valuable. Similarly, within scheme two, the need for facilitators to be committed to focusing on the process of the group emerged as a key theme. This meant viewing group members as a powerful resource, just as important as any content which might be delivered within the session itself. In order to embrace this principle, it was seen as important for the facilitator to invest time at the beginning of any IPL session in allowing the group to form their own identity and establish ground rules. In the evidence from the Delphi survey it was clearly demonstrated that diverse IPL groups, by their very nature, consist of individuals who bring with them a whole host of past experiences, work and professional issues, expectations and different learning styles. As a result, this process can be fraught with difficulties and may become uncomfortable.

Facilitators are therefore required to understand group dynamics, have the courage to handle this purposefully and acquire skills for managing group tension and conflict constructively. Basic skills about managing group dynamics may be acquired. Much has already been written about this but facilitators who engage in formative evaluation and reflective practice will be able to hone these skills further.

Managing issues around power and hierarchy

Issues around power and hierarchy were raised and discussed at considerable length within schemes two and three, suggesting that they play a significant part in IPL. The unequal power base which may be present amongst group members in an IPL session and the effect of professional stereotyping within IPL groups were identified as issues of which facilitators must be acutely aware. In addition it was seen as crucial that facilitators should be aware of their own power within the group through their own professional background but also by virtue of their position as group facilitator.

Scheme one demonstrated that power can be exerted not merely from professionals themselves, but by professional governing and accrediting bodies. The original aim for this scheme was to develop and evaluate the course for GP trainers as an interprofessional course and introduce interprofessional teaching. A small number of other professionals joined the course and thus offered the potential for it to become interprofessional. There were however several problems, such as the other professionals unable to assess the GPs and the status of GP trainer, a role not open to other professionals. The main benefit of the change was to that of an interprofessional teaching team with the emphasis on an increased focus on generic teaching skills and a tutor team who were able to reflect the values of IPL. Attitudes of GP trainers emerging from the revised programme now reflect the values of IPL to a greater degree than before the intervention. This is evidenced by their plans to draw on the expertise of other professionals in their practices, when devising educational programmes for GP registrars.

Although, there has been some shift towards IPL values at the course level and by the teaching teams, the power exerted by the professional governing bodies makes change to an interprofessional course unlikely at present. This is an area which needs to be acknowledged by facilitators of IPL and explored within IPL activities, power has great significance and occurs at many different levels.

The result of power differentials and of professional stereotypes not being reconciled was very apparent within the interview transcripts analysed in scheme two. The 'language of war and conflict' was used throughout by participants when referring to other professional groups and interprofessional relationships. Having the means to explore and manage issues around power and hierarchy therefore emerged as an essential component for successful IPL.

It would appear therefore, that anyone undertaking IPL facilitation, who lacks appreciation and awareness of the role of power within complex, diverse groups, does so at their peril. Failure to acknowledge the significance of power and hierarchies within a mixed professional group may result in failure to achieve the level of trust required for all the group members to be able to participate fully. Not only is this an opportunity lost, it could create or reinforce negative assumptions and beliefs about other professionals which then become hidden deep within the iceberg of professional practice.

Planning IPL

The fifth theme, which emerged strongly from the research undertaken within scheme three and four, was the need to address the context in which any IPL occurs. Gaining advance information about the participants, their backgrounds and giving some thought to existing contentious issues which participants might bring into the IPL setting with them were viewed as important. Equally essential, was the awareness of external factors which may impact on learning such as organisational structures, policies and procedures. This issue was clearly illustrated within scheme one, where the significance of the influence of external forces such as work pressures for certain professionals and constraints from the GP training standards body were underestimated with regards to developing a truly interprofessional generic teaching skills programme. If facilitators are unaware of such important issues, it is very difficult for them to relate learning to the realities of the work environment and the process could lack authenticity. Indeed, some of the students in the focus groups cited having the opportunity to relate classroom teaching to the realities of the work environment as an essential component of IPL. The need to pay equal attention to the content and process of the IPL educational event was particularly highlighted in scheme four where IPL seminars in health inequalities were being piloted. Gaining the commitment of all the participating organisations in order that the IPL was a truly collaborative activity was also viewed as important. The issues relevant to this are explored further in Chapter 7. Finally, the need to give attention to the learning environment, specifically, practical details such as the room being an appropriate size with the ability to move chairs around and arrangements for refreshments was highlighted.

This attention to context and relevance reflects a particular value which, we would suggest, is fundamental to any teaching situation, i.e. the duty of care to all learners, both in terms of comfort and respect for ensuring time well spent on a learning activity that would be relevant and applicable back at base. IPL facilitators need to invest time in these aspects so that this value may be experienced. They should also have thought in advance about how to deal with difficult situations which might arise.

The facilitator's learning philosophy

An important finding which strongly emerged from scheme two was that successful facilitators tend to have a particular philosophy of learning and indeed of life in general, not just to IPL. This philosophy encompasses a commitment to the beliefs and values of adult learning and inclusivity. It is reflected in the way they view the world and the way they value others as individuals. Such values are clearly integral to their teaching processes and the way in which these values are modelled is an issue which requires careful consideration on the part of the facilitator.

It is clearly impossible to 'teach' this in any formal sense, but such an approach to learning may be fostered and nurtured in a number of ways. Firstly, through role modelling of those from whom they learn facilitation. Secondly, the opportunity to co-facilitate with others means that there is not only back-up and the chance to take turns at adopting a forward or backward role throughout the event, but also an opportunity for the co-facilitators to provide each other with feedback. Thirdly, inviting other peers to observe and provide constructive feedback helps facilitators to stay open to development and learning themselves. It should be the established practice of any person involved in teaching, training or facilitation to receive peer observation on a regular basis. At present, although this often occurs within higher education, it is far less frequent within practice environments. It is something we would suggest is vital for all facilitators to undertake. An appropriate person (i.e. someone who will provide an objective, constructively critical view of the facilitator) should be identified to attend a session purely as an observer and not as a participant. This activity should occur at least annually and more frequently in the case of newly appointed IPL facilitators.

IPL facilitators who have themselves engaged in experiential learning within IPL groups will find it easier to understand and accept that IPL facilitation is usually complex and unpredictable. They may be less likely to blame themselves for any difficult experience but be more open to the need for learning and development through these. Certainly, one of the outcomes of scheme one was that attitudes of the GP trainers emerging from the revised programme with a wider professional mix of both students and members of the teaching team, reflected the values of IPL to a greater degree. The work of scheme four demonstrated the value of being part of a learner set for IPL facilitators. Over the course of the project, this provided a safe forum for sharing problematic issues in running IPL events, celebrating IPL successes and even a setting in which interprofessional tensions and resolutions could be played out because the participants of scheme four were, themselves, interprofessional in constitution. In scheme one, the opportunity to engage in an IPL team at a programme planning level was considered to be very valuable in terms of widening the perspectives of the teaching team and subsequently, the students on the programme.

The discussion on the six themes of facilitator preparation which emerged from the whole of the PIPE project offer many ideas, suggestions and a value base on which to help facilitators prepare for their role. One way that some of these themes have been put into practice can be found in the following example (Box 5.2) which sets out how two of the PIPE project team members built the experience of IPL into a workshop on group facilitation skills.

The next section builds on this practical application of how facilitation can be learnt in practice and offers some realistic suggestions.

Learning and developing facilitation skills in practice

Institutions and communities of educators need to acknowledge that IPL facilitation is a complex activity. At the institutional level, there needs to be commitment not to throw the 'rookie' teacher in at the deep end without support. Any person beginning a role involving facilitating interprofessional groups should be encouraged to develop a personal 'programme' of experiential and learning activities, to support their personal and professional growth during their first year in the post.

A philosophy of nurturing and supporting people into new roles is at the very core of the National Health Service (NHS) Knowledge and Skills Framework[13] which provides a useful model for how this could be achieved. The novice facilitator would consider the demands and requirements of their role and 'match' their existing knowledge, skills and abilities against these. They would then produce a personal development plan identifying learning and development needs, set goals and then create a plan for how they could achieve these goals. They would be encouraged to learn and develop their facilitation skills in a variety of ways with the support of an experienced facilitator. Examples could be:

BOX 5.2 Developing skills in facilitating complex, diverse groups: learning through working as an interprofessional group

Two of the PIPE team members work in primary care and were approached by managers from some of the local primary care trusts. They were concerned about the lack of experience that some of the specialist nurses and other healthcare professionals had in undertaking the training and group facilitation which was a key aspect of their roles. The PIPE team members agreed to run two workshops in order to enable such professionals to develop their skills in facilitating interprofessional learning. When the workshops were advertised the response was overwhelming. Whereas it was expected that a small number of mainly specialist nurses would apply, in fact, a large number of people from a wide variety of professional, training and support roles did so. This appeared to support the starting premise of the PIPE three project, that there are large numbers of staff within the workplace facilitating complex, diverse groups who require additional levels of knowledge, skills and experience. It also became apparent that in addition to the variety of professional backgrounds there was also a rich mix among the delegates in terms of race, nationality, gender and age.

The PIPE members considered this to be a great opportunity to enable the participants to learn and develop their skills primarily through the experience of working within diverse groups. The workshops therefore consisted of a series of group activities exploring different aspects of group facilitation. Such activities included producing drawings depicting a facilitator and a trainer, discussing strategies for dealing with challenging situations during IPL sessions and identifying types of behaviour from group participants which might trigger personal emotional responses from themselves. After each activity, the participants were asked to feed back the results to the other groups and also to reflect on their experiences of the process, particularly with regards to the impact of their own values, beliefs and assumptions. They were also required to 'regroup' several times throughout the day, thus enabling them to experience different group dynamics. The group activities were interspersed with presentations on different theories of facilitation and findings from the PIPE project.

The workshops were thus structured in a way which enabled the participants to experience and explore the emotional and social/environmental aspects of learning as well as the cognitive. The feedback from the workshops was extremely positive and the participants clearly valued the opportunity to be able to learn and develop their skills in this way.

- shadowing experienced IPL facilitators: this would allow observation of the aspects of professional practice that experienced IPL facilitators demonstrate which are less explicit and which they may find difficult to articulate. The novice facilitator would be encouraged to evaluate the teaching practice observed and then reflect upon and analyse this with the experienced facilitator at the end of the session

- co-facilitation and buddy teaching: this requires specific preparation in terms of negotiating the division of leadership and responsibilities within the session, styles of facilitation, how to deal with issues that may arise, etc. The novice facilitator could initially take a less active role in facilitating sessions but gradually become more actively involved as their level of knowledge and skills develop. This would enable them to gain confidence in their ability over a period of time
- opportunity to engage in formative evaluation of IPL activity: this promotes critical thinking about the process and effect of IPL activities
- opportunity for mentoring: this provides protected time and attention with another teacher for reflection within a safe environment
- opportunity for engaging in learner sets: similar opportunity for reflection as in mentoring but, in addition, it provides the support and collaborative learning of a peer group. As we have indicated, IPL is inherently complex and it is particularly valuable for facilitators to have the opportunity to 'pool' a range of ideas for improving their skills and dealing with difficult issues which may arise during the process
- opportunity for engaging in interprofessional programme planning teams: provides opportunity for experiencing interprofessional activity and influencing the way in which interprofessional learning develops.

Individuals would be required to evaluate this programme of learning and development, identify how they were applying it to their teaching practice and demonstrate professional growth.

Although such activities are particularly important in the first year, acknowledgement of the complex, dynamic nature of facilitating interprofessional learning, institutions, organisations and individuals themselves need to accept that facilitators of IPL will never become 'experts' – they will need to continue to review and develop their skills for as long as they remain in such roles.

Conclusion

Interprofessional interactions are, by their very nature, dynamic and spontaneous, and impossible to choreograph. Learning to facilitate IPL cannot therefore be achieved by undertaking a prescribed course or programme. However, it is perfectly possible to rehearse situations and scenarios, learn from experience and seek to broaden the base of the iceberg of professional practice and strengthen its foundations. For the purposes of this chapter, we assumed that IPL facilitators are already knowledgeable about the content of the learning. We considered how they might prepare themselves to help their students in the other dimensions of learning: emotional processes and interaction with the world around them.

The evidence from all of the PIPE schemes has implications for the process of preparing facilitators for IPL or, indeed, for facilitating any complex diverse groups. Facilitators need to be self-aware:

- to be able to deal with difference and conflict
- to understand group processes and relationships
- to be able to handle power issues
- to be based on real patient/carer isssues
- to plan carefully for the context of learning.

This may sound like a daunting prospect, even for experienced teachers, but we would argue that many teachers and facilitators already hold much of this explicit and tacit knowledge within themselves. They simply need help, support and opportunities to gain this awareness and deepen their understanding. In short, facilitation of IPL should be undertaken within the structured, reflective framework which we advocated earlier in the chapter. Without the proper support and investment in this, IPL facilitators would be, at best, ineffective and at worst, counter-productive. We would argue that it is only through fully engaging in the reflective process and developing higher level skills in this area, that practitioners are able to successfully role model the attitude that is necessary for effective interprofessional learning and working to occur. With the right preparation, IPL facilitators can help their learners to unlock the potential within themselves. The most important factor is time, space and willingness to reflect upon and unpick one's own practice, attitudes, beliefs and values, within a supportive environment. Fundamentally, this requires a personal commitment and institutional support.

The values of interprofessional learning need to be similarly reflected in curricula development, so that the facilitation process is matched by an appropriate context, in which interprofessional learning may flourish. Curricula development and the role of the institutions in enabling such environments are discussed in the next chapter.

CHAPTER 6

Curriculum development for interprofessional learning

MAGGIE LORD AND GILL YOUNG

Introduction

This chapter will examine how curricula can be developed to prepare teachers and facilitators to teach interprofessional groups. Although the evidence base for interprofessional working continues to grow, there is little published material on how teachers or facilitators should be prepared to teach interprofessional learning. Evidence from the PIPE project will be used to discuss different curricula approaches for the preparation of teachers for interprofessional learning. The decision to use the 'evolution' curriculum to incorporate a common learning outcome used by four different higher education institutions will be explored. Evaluation and comparison of the impact on curriculum development will be presented using a sustainable interprofessional learning framework.

The chapter will begin by offering an exploration of the term 'curriculum', emphasising the complexity of selecting frameworks for teaching and learning which have been presented in Chapter 2 of this book and the complexity of selecting approaches to curriculum development in all disciplines, as well as those in health and social care. The impact of influences and motives for interprofessional learning on the outcomes of curriculum development will be evaluated and the chapter will conclude by presenting conditions that influence and lead to curriculum development for successful interprofessional learning and education.

What does the term 'curriculum' mean?

Academic disciplines are underpinned by different and often distinct understandings of what constitutes knowledge and of the appropriate ways to approach teaching, learning and, importantly, curriculum development. Even within the same discipline or profession, courses have discrete cultures and influences, therefore attempting to define the curriculum may be contentious. A study of the literature confirms that as a concept, curriculum is difficult to define. There are many definitions of curriculum and interpretation of the term has created uncertainty.[1] Kelly[2] claims that knowledge of curriculum studies has diminished in the UK and relates this to the influence of governmental initiatives influencing education policy. The influence of the political desire for interprofessional working has had a similar effect on curriculum development in health and social care in the UK. This political motive is becoming prevalent in the majority of healthcare systems worldwide although curriculum textbooks from other continents may provide diverse approaches to definitions or guidance. For example Uys and Gwele[3] are from South Africa and their recent book still makes reference to a uniprofessional nursing context. Iwasiw *et al*[1] are from the USA where the approach to curriculum planning is still about long-term and whole curriculum development.

Kelly[2] critiques the present day curriculum as focusing on content and product rather than on process and development and is highly critical of the way the study of curriculum theory has been developed in the UK over the last 20 years. Neary[4] identifies two main approaches to defining the curriculum. The first approach emphasises the overall plans and intentions of the educators. In this approach the curriculum can be defined as the formulation and implementation of an educational proposal and is at the collective level. Neary's second approach to curriculum focuses on what individual teachers do in the classroom or on the skills and knowledge of the learners, whether this learning is intended or not. In this approach, the curriculum can broadly be seen as a statement of what counts as knowledge, embracing the students' engagement with the offering put before them. The curriculum also defines the learning outcomes or objectives, educational content and sequencing, the characteristics of the learning experiences especially the methods and mode to be used, the resources for teaching and learning, where teaching will take place, the assessment methods, and how the programme will be evaluated. Thus the curriculum is a complex of interrelated processes where changing one aspect will lead to changes in others.[5] There have been changes in the overall view of the curriculum and curriculum development in recent years.

These changes are:
- recognition of the importance of the process of learning as well as the outcomes or learning products[4]
- a greater emphasis on the active participation of the learner in the learning process
- a greater emphasis on the context in which teaching and learning take place
- a growing differentiation between the roles of teacher as opposed to the facilitator of a group.

These changes are evident in Chapters 3 and 4 of this book, where knowledge and awareness of context and group processes are essential for the educator.

The development of a curriculum does not take place in a vacuum: it is influenced by factors within the institution such as quality assurance mechanisms, teaching, learning and assessment strategies, and external factors such as statutory and professional body requirements. But it is also influenced by less definable factors such as the characteristics, pedagogical beliefs and ideas of the development team members, and their perception of the students' needs. These latter, being individually held, are often the most difficult factors for curriculum team members to articulate, understand, and reach agreement on, during both curriculum development and delivery. These lead to competing demands on and for the curriculum. Awareness of these factors is vital whether producing a curriculum for a whole course, a module or short course, a workshop or a single session. They should include knowledge of the appropriateness of teaching methods, for example the principles of demonstrations, workshops or facilitation. In a curriculum for teacher preparation, this needs to include experience and practice of these approaches.

Curriculum development approaches for interprofessional learning

All the factors mentioned above are magnified when developing an interprofessional curriculum. This was clearly demonstrated by one student teacher when being interviewed for the PIPE scheme two research:

> ...in my experience, people genuinely are open to the notion of putting different student groups together. What prevents it often is the curriculum, and time and resources.

Since interprofessional education is a fairly new approach, especially in undergraduate education, there is no tried and tested model to guide development. There is ongoing discourse and debate about the most appropriate time for interprofessional education to occur: this is outlined in Chapter 1 which asks whether interprofessional learning should be introduced at the undergraduate or pre-qualifying stage or whether an individual first needs to be comfortable with their own professional identify before being able to engage with the notion of the identities of others.[6] This is evidenced by the following statement from the PIPE research project:

> I don't know, I think there's a big question as well, because we're mixing pre- and post-registration students, on one hand it seems that pre-registration students need to identify a uniprofessional identity for us to deconstruct it and that seems quite interesting that somebody needs to have a feeling of who they are before you can actually challenge who they think they are.

Two broad approaches have emerged in this decade which can be characterised as revolution and evolution. The revolution model is characterised by the creation of a new interprofessional curriculum with timetabled shared learning, teaching and assessment elements in both classroom and practice settings. This revolution curriculum approach to interprofessional learning involves major change for all the professions, institutions, teachers and students involved, major resources both financial and human, to project manage its development and delivery. An example of this model would be Southampton and Portsmouth Universities' New Generation project.[7]

The second approach which can be labelled as evolution is characterised by incremental changes to existing curricula. Institutions and professions work collaboratively to gradually move to the position outlined above in the revolution model. This usually commences with the incorporation of common learning outcomes into all programmes which will be summatively assessed, but often by different methods in each of the curricula. This also requires both financial and human resources to implement, especially providing all students with interprofessional learning experiences in undergraduate programmes with their large student numbers, but less than the revolutionary model. This approach has been developed particularly where there are many institutions involved with little or no previous history of collaboration in learning and teaching. An example of this approach is the collaborative interprofessional learning programme developed in North West London formally known as the Joint Universities Multiprofessional Programme (JUMP).[8] In this geographical area, students from individual professions are taught in several higher education institutions. In order to experience shared or interprofessional learning, the students are brought together, while on placement, to work together on a shared enquiry based learning scenario with facilitators from the placement trusts.

It is this evolutionary model which has also been used in the PIPE project by the four universities which have postgraduate teacher preparation programmes. The four institutions had no history of collaboration in this aspect of postgraduate provision, and were competitors for students for these programmes. This is always a factor in inter-institutional collaboration, but more so in programmes such as these which are largely or entirely outside the National Health Service contracts for educational provision. The reasons why the four universities involved in the scheme chose to collaborate are discussed in Chapter 7. It is important to note, that for such collaboration to be successful, the project had to meet each of the institutions' individual objectives.

It was apparent to the collaborators in the PIPE two scheme that, although there was literature evaluating evidence in this area of interprofessional work, there was a dearth of evidence relating to interdisciplinary teacher preparation for interprofessional education. The description and analysis of this aspect of the PIPE scheme is complex. Four higher education institutions were involved in the scheme, each with its own culture, bureaucracy and experience of interprofessional learning and teaching. Each was starting from a unique position and each would have a different outcome. With little educational research to support major curricula change, and insufficient resources, both financial and human, to use the revolutionary approach, the PIPE scheme team had to achieve consensus and a common approach. It has to be remembered that the students on these programmes were already experienced in their own professions or disciplines, and each of the curricula for teacher preparation had evolved in their own contexts over a period of time. Initially the starting positions of the different institutions were mapped and the possibilities for change explored, such as whether an existing, successful, module from one institution could be incorporated into the other programmes. It was evident that, as the universities had different structures, this would not be possible and the most achievable objective was to develop and incorporate a common learning outcome for interprofessional leaning. This outcome was then incorporated and evaluated within the four programmes. The common learning outcome was framed as:

> Students will explore opportunities for interprofessional collaboration which influence or lead to informal/formal learning.

The evaluation of the scheme included research into the experiences of the students and programme teams. This is presented in depth in Chapter 4. The overall impact of involvement in the PIPE project and schemes was also discussed following the analysis of the findings of this evaluation. One of the strengths of the project was that the project and scheme teams were made up of academics and professionals with a wealth of experience and knowledge of the field of professional and adult education. This was linked with enthusiasm and led to wide-ranging discussion of new approaches and frameworks, mixing scholarship from different fields where it seemed appropriate. Developing an approach that would enhance the likelihood of embedding interprofessional learning into the programmes was discussed, and a framework to present this was then prepared.

How the universities incorporated the common learning outcome

Each of the institutions incorporated the learning outcome differently. For one university, this meant major change, membership of the PIPE project being one of the motives behind this change. The institution had previously had an MA in Learning and Teaching offered only to nursing and midwifery lecturers and practice educators from their partner NHS trusts based in the Faculty of Health and Human Sciences. This was a postgraduate certificate programme being run centrally in the university to enable new lecturers to meet the Higher Education Academy's requirements. The incorporation of the PIPE (scheme two) learning outcome into the curriculum coincided with a major review of teacher preparation in the university and the design of a new MA in Learning and Teaching. This brought the two together to provide a new interprofessional, interdisciplinary teacher preparation programme for all new lecturers and practice educators. As part of the new programme a new ten credit module was designed with the title of 'interprofessional education'. This module was designed to be delivered by e-learning using Blackboard version 5.0 and later version 6.0. Evidence and expert input from the JUMP project,[8] of which the university was a member, and from PIPE, were incorporated into the materials. The decision to use electronic delivery was partly driven by the need to be able to update materials rapidly as this field was developing so fast.

This major change also enabled the designers to use the PIPE learning outcome as a focus for the module's assessment of learning. The students being required to organise, deliver and evaluate an interprofessional learning event. Evidence from the first cohort's assignments indicated that the introduction of the PIPE learning outcome was very successful, leading in many cases to the beginnings of sustained interprofessional learning for the teachers.

In the second university, incorporating the PIPE learning outcome brought about a move from little explicit focus on interprofessional learning being in the programme, to it being an integral component, addressed not in a discrete module but threaded through the programme. The mix of students on the programme has also become increasingly diverse. Groupwork and seminars were organised to enable students to learn about, with and from other professions, and to critically debate issues in interprofessional learning. There was also a change in the students' teaching practice and assignments which incorporated an interprofessional learning perspective. The organisation of the content relating to interprofessional learning was delivered as a series of workshop days.

The third institution had a programme leading to an MA in Education with a series of intermediate awards. This led to a qualification in education that can be recorded with the relevant statutory body and leads to membership of the Higher Education Academy. The students on this programme were either nurses, midwives or specialist community practice nurses who were lecturers in the institution or working as practice or clinical educators in the local trusts. The course was run in parallel with the in-house course for lecturers in other disciplines in the institution. There were opportunities for interdisciplinary and shared sessions between the groups. In this programme the learning outcome was addressed as a theme throughout the course and incorporated into the relevant modules. Many of the students on the programme were involved in teaching interprofessional groups in practice and in curriculum development with other professions for study days on topics such as child protection.

At the fourth institution there was a well-developed programme leading to an MSc in Education with a series of intermediate awards. The participants on the programme came from the range of professions represented in the institution. A commitment to interprofessional education was already integrated into this programme and the students undertook two modules relevant to interprofessional learning: a group process and facilitation skills module and a module dedicated to interprofessional education. It was initially hoped that these modules could be incorporated into the other programmes. However, structures in higher education do not easily lend themselves to such rapid change and, as previously stated, only the change that could be implemented across all programmes was made.

Evaluating the impact of PIPE involvement on the programmes and curriculum teams

Evaluation of the effects of a complex problem was not unique to the PIPE project. Church and Shouldice[9] point out that evaluation is an ad hoc process conforming to the needs of the moment and limited by lack of skills, understanding and resources. In social programmes change is influenced by multiple layers[10] and identifying and accounting for these layers was a challenge. Kirkpatrick's model of evaluating teacher performance on training courses identifies a hierarchy of four levels of evaluation:[11]

- level one which is reaction. This asks participants how they feel about the various aspects of training programmes. However, this can be perceived as being subjective, reflecting whether or not participants enjoyed the experience
- level two which reflects what the participants have learned from the experience. This focuses on whether the participants have acquired knowledge, improved their skills or changed their attitudes changed as a result of training. However, this again is self reported and subjective
- level three is about behaviour and tries to reflect a measure of how participants change their on-the-job behaviour as a result of training and may be assessed after three months
- level four is about results. These may be about reducing costs, improving quality or productivity and lowering absenteeism and turnover.

It is these examples of valuing the product of training rather than the process of education which are critiqued by Kelly.[2] These are some of the pedagogical beliefs and ideas that curriculum development teams need to debate during the development process. In the PIPE two scheme, one way of evaluating the impact of incorporating the learning outcome was by using focus groups to elicit views from the students and programme teams at the end of the implementation phase. An in-depth account of this evaluation of reaction has been provided in Chapter 4, but the wider effect and the outcomes in the institutions needed to be framed to allow comparison of the impact on each. At the beginning there were four institutions, four positions, four baselines and, following the implementation, four changed positions. A framework to demonstrate the changes and allow comparisons of complex outcomes was needed. Ways of presenting these changes were debated, identifying pre-existing evaluation research to inform the development of practice.

A framework for evaluating PIPE scheme two interventions was developed by loosely combining other frameworks: one for the evaluation of conflict resolution interventions[9] which outlines the intervention and outcomes of the project, and one for sustainable livelihoods [12] which was used to frame the likelihood of sustaining the PIPE initiative into future programmes.

Church and Shouldice[9] proposed a conflict-specific framework which could integrate the different aspects of an intervention that can be evaluated. This was structured round three themes:

- goals and interventions: which explore the use of (conflict) analysis when planning an intervention and the theoretical and ideological basis of an organisation's strategy. This element asks the question, 'why and how is the agency conducting this intervention?'
- process: this assesses the implementation of an intervention. This theme asks, 'how was the intervention put into place?'

■ range of results: this considers the results achieved through the intervention. This theme asks, 'what were the short-term and long-term results of the intervention?'

These were easily related to the aim and implementation of PIPE scheme two which was to improve the preparation of future teachers by enhancing the provision of postgraduate interprofessional learning programmes for teachers in higher education. The process of evaluation has been described in Chapter 4 but the range of outcomes will be presented later in this chapter. Two additional concepts to inform the discussion are the tiers of influence,[9] and the focus of change.[9]

The tiers of influence,[9] consider who an intervention is targeting. In the PIPE context this relates to individual students and programme teams but there is also a ripple effect and an intervention might influence peer group, community or future students. This is illuminated by the following statement:

> And almost I think teachers are the top end of that. So if you can teach the teachers who then go out and teach professionals, who will then go forward and hopefully have some of these values, then that, I think, is a really good place to start.

The focus of change[9] addresses what an interaction is seeking to influence and this is more complex as the influence does not have to be limited to one level as depending on the scope of the interventions and a number of levels could be relevant. These could include: the broad social and political environment; structures and institutions; approaches and procedures; physical/financial; behaviours and skills or attitudes and beliefs,[9] all of which are relevant in the PIPE context. For example, Chapter 1 gives an account of the social and political context of the whole project and Chapter 3 explores the skills required by facilitators.

These additional themes can also be blended with a framework used in international development which looks at the elements of sustainable systems including social and institutional sustainability.[13] These frameworks were appropriate because they recognise complex systems and recognise multiple influences, strategies and diverse outcomes. These systems are seen to accumulate stocks of assets and it is these assets that are of most interest.[9,12] These livelihoods are dynamic, complex, and subject to external forces for example social, economic, political, or institutional.[14] These reflect some of the complexities encountered in the PIPE project. Additionally the framework can be represented pictorially which made it easy to use and display for discussion (*see* Figure 6.1).

PIPE sustainable interprofessional learning framework baseline comparisons

Elements from the frameworks were adapted for the PIPE scheme. The areas for evaluation focused on:

■ the original context

PIPE two interventions: baselines

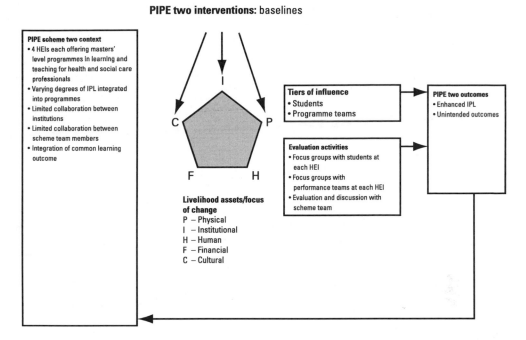

FIGURE 6.1 Sustainable frameworks. Based on Chambers and Conway (1991) and Church and Shouldice (2002).

- the intervention
- the activities developed
- the tiers of influence which affect these activities
- the outcomes of the intervention
- the focus of change related to the cultural, human, financial, social, and institutional assets.

Each institution began with a baseline description of relevant activities at the beginning of the project when the learning outcome was introduced; this is represented in Figure 6.1.

These were reviewed at the end of the project, focusing on the institutional context, the tiers of influence over the intervention, the barriers to embedding the change, the outcomes of the intervention and the assets to the institution of being involved in the PIPE project including changes to courses particularly those which made the courses more similar.

Evaluation of the impact of PIPE involvement on the programmes and curriculum teams

At the end of the project each of the teams presented the changes to their programmes based on the sustainable interprofessional learning framework (Figure 6.2). Where the

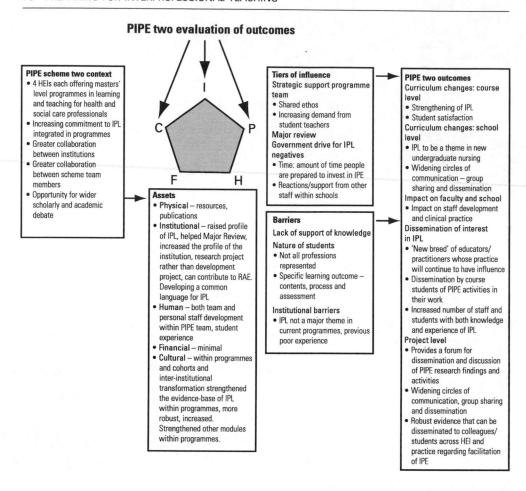

PIPE two evaluation of outcomes

PIPE scheme two context
- 4 HEIs each offering masters' level programmes in learning and teaching for health and social care professionals
- Increasing commitment to IPL integrated in programmes
- Greater collaboration between institutions
- Greater collaboration between scheme team members
- Opportunity for wider scholarly and academic debate

I
C P
F H

Assets
- **Physical** – resources, publications
- **Institutional** – raised profile of IPL, helped Major Review, increased the profile of the institution, research project rather than development project, can contribute to RAE. Developing a common language for IPL
- **Human** – both team and personal staff development within PIPE team, student experience
- **Financial** – minimal
- **Cultural** – within programmes and cohorts and inter-institutional transformation strengthened the evidence-base of IPL within programmes, more robust, increased. Strengthened other modules within programmes.

Tiers of influence
Strategic support programme team
- Shared ethos
- Increasing demand from student teachers

Major review
Government drive for IPL
negatives
- Time: amount of time people are prepared to invest in IPE
- Reactions/support from other staff within schools

Barriers
Lack of support of knowledge
Nature of students
- Not all professions represented
- Specific learning outcome – contents, process and assessment

Institutional barriers
- IPL not a major theme in current programmes, previous poor experience

PIPE two outcomes
Curriculum changes: course level
- Strengthening of IPL
- Student satisfaction
Curriculum changes: school level
- IPL to be a theme in new undergraduate nursing
- Widening circles of communication – group sharing and dissemination
Impact on faculty and school
- Impact on staff development and clinical practice
Dissemination of interest in IPL
- 'New breed' of educators/ practitioners whose practice will continue to have influence
- Dissemination by course students of PIPE activities in their work
- Increased number of staff and students with both knowledge and experience of IPL
Project level
- Provides a forum for dissemination and discussion of PIPE research findings and activities
- Widening circles of communication, group sharing and dissemination
- Robust evidence that can be disseminated to colleagues/ students across HEI and practice regarding facilitation of IPE

FIGURE 6.2 PIPE sustainable IPL frameworks. Based on Chambers and Conway (1991) and Church and Shouldice (2002).

activities had been implemented, the barriers to the implementation took the place of the activities element. The curriculum development undertaken in the relevant programme can not be seen as taking place in a vacuum. The activities undertaken within each institution affected and were therefore absorbed into the outcomes. This section will provide an overview based around the barriers, assets, tiers of influence and outcomes. The tiers of influence, which occur at different levels, could lead to influences which could be positive or negative and where there was resistance at one level, this could pose a barrier. These influences have therefore been presented in the same themes.

Tiers of influence
These influences occurred at different levels. These important factors which were common to all programmes were strategic influences, support, the nature of the students and specific aspects related to individual programmes.

Strategic support

A positive influence for all programmes came from implicit strategic support. All of the programmes were to be reviewed for ongoing quality monitoring by the UK Quality Assurance Agency (QAA). One area to be tested was ongoing commitment to interprofessional learning and involvement in the PIPE project was universally viewed as a positive influence. This also held true for the UK government initiative for interprofessional working and learning and the efforts of the funding bodies or strategic health authorities to promote this. The JUMP[8] project is an example of this as it was an initiative directly funded by one workforce development confederation. The requirements of the professional awarding bodies such as the Nursing and Midwifery Council and the Higher Education Academy's teacher standards were also enhanced across the programmes by the focus on interprofessional learning.

Support

While this level of support from the Strategic Health Authorities' Clinical Trust Directors was important, the support within the programmes and programme teams was paramount. This varied between the programmes and was linked in part to stability or instability in the programme teams. A shared ethos and approach to teaching and learning was seen as constructive which was evidenced through the focus groups. The programme teams were also able to have discussion about the nature of student learning which was seen as positive. Where the professions were taught together and taught by an interprofessional programme team, this could help with modelling of interprofessional values.

Nature of students

Not all programmes involved more than one profession and no programme had all the professions present. The time required to implement the project and enhance interprofessional education was seen as demanding, however the increasing interest and even demand from the student teachers to be more prepared to facilitate interprofessional learning justified this. Where faculties or schools supported the time dedicated to IPL or had a community of resources available, this was helpful. However in one institution the reaction of other staff to the project member was negative and unsupportive. Here, the support of the project team was especially helpful.

Barriers

These can be discussed within similar categories as the tiers of influence as there is the potential for these elements to be either positive or negative.

Lack of support

One barrier was the amount of time and the quantity of work expended by the PIPE scheme two representative during the evaluation phase. This was not always seen as a valuable use of time by other faculty members: even where it was seen as legitimate, it was still time consuming for all the project members. Another barrier was lack of knowledge and continuing professional development in educational development among higher education staff. Although lecturing staff maintain current knowledge in their clinical or academic field, updating in teaching and learning issues is seen as a lesser priority. This means that assumptions are made and the debate about acknowledging interprofessional learning opportunities across a range of settings is limited. This was reinforced by the fact that education is often viewed as low priority within healthcare trusts and in financial crises it is often the first thing to be rationalised. This lack of value placed on the work varied between institutions and at different times.

Nature of students

As these programmes are for teacher preparation, there are relatively low numbers of students on them compared to other programmes. This put their continuity under threat as they were seen as non-viable by managers in the long term. There was also the problem of the limited range of professional backgrounds of students across some of the programmes as many were uniprofessional in years two and three of a programme. Another barrier was the funding issue since different funding bodies had differing funding streams for medical education and non-medical education and training (NMET). Although there was funding in place for some students, they had difficulty in being released from the workplace for the required study days. This affected the group process and the ability to explore issues such as professional power and identity.

Programme team issues

Introducing a new learning outcome into existing programmes meant changes in process, content and assessment. Due to the nature of the programmes, the teaching teams were experienced lecturers and taught on accredited programmes both nationally and internationally. They therefore had developed views about pedagogical issues. Where only certain members of the team were involved in the project, this meant that they had to work harder to influence the whole programme. This made change to the programmes more difficult, especially since it involved a change in approach and values rather than just updating content.

Strategic influences

An ongoing influence from the professional bodies, was their growing role in public protection and their decreasing role in providing a consistent approach for the requirements of teachers of professionals.

Institutional barriers

Interprofessional learning is not a major theme in most current undergraduate or postgraduate programmes and, although this is gradually changing, this means that there are few lecturers, lecturer practitioners and practice educators with experience and knowledge of facilitating interprofessional learning. Those that have experience may not have had preparation in teaching and learning or facilitating groups, and few have had specific preparation for facilitating interprofessional groups. In some instances there was a tension between the value placed on the content of interprofessional learning which was seen as less demanding than teaching expert and specialist knowledge. Often it is the lecturer new to higher education who is asked to facilitate interprofessional learning. The turnover of staff in the institutions during the PIPE project also had an impact. In some instances there was little will to promote IPL among individuals as it was not seen as a priority in the overall work of faculties or schools. Some staff had previous poor experience of being involved in interprofessional working and learning or were critical of the UK government's intentions.

Assets
These are essential for sustaining the impetus generated by being part of the project. There was much agreement among the institutions for these assets.

Physical
All the institutions have gained physical resources such as a wider range of readings in the learning resource centre, the increased range of academic texts made available to the students. Programme team members from other institutions were able to teach on the other programmes. One institution also has an e-learning module.

Institutional
In all of the institutions being involved in the project they were helped both in major quality reviews and in the development of new pre-registration curricula where many of the student teachers were able to contribute more fully. Being involved in the project also increased the profile of interprofessional learning in the faculties or schools and throughout the universities and also raised the profile of the institutions involved in the project beyond the participating universities. The project supported interprofessional learning development for undergraduate students initiated through the JUMP programme, where some of the practice educator students were facilitators for this initiative. The fact that the project was a publicly-funded research project rather than a development project was also a benefit for the institutions involved, where inter-institutional research is rated highly.

Human
The human assets emanating from the project were immense. The student experience of interprofessional learning improved and many took part in workshops and activities organised through the project. In one instance the programme team and students worked together to develop an e-learning programme. There was also a remarkable amount of personal staff development within the PIPE team, which was highly valued and achieved as a result of the project.

Financial
In all of the institutions there has been an increased short-term input. The expenditure has been minimal beyond normal new module development costs. This

should not affect the future sustainability of the impetus for interprofessional learning.

Cultural

Within the programmes the importance of, and impetus for, developing an approach to interprofessional education rooted in the PIPE project outcomes had been developed to different extents in the institutions. In two of the institutions this has been overwhelmingly positive, while it has been less so in two others. The positive effects have been a combination of introducing interprofessional education/interprofessional learning as major themes in the programme, and strengthening the evidence-base of interprofessional learning. Other modules have also been strengthened within other programmes. Assessments are more frequently related to aspects of interprofessional learning and there have been increased educational events in university and practice. The attitude to the value of collaboration with other institutions has been transformed. However, in two of the institutions, there has been a more limited effect especially in the wider school or faculty mainly due to changes in staff since commencement of the project and in one institution resulting in the overall culture within the school.

PIPE scheme two outcomes

However, it is in the programme outcomes where the most valuable work has been done and changes have been seen. These can be described under the headings of curriculum changes, impact on the schools, project level changes, and outcomes beyond the project.

Curriculum changes: course level

There was increased uptake of students choosing interprofessional learning as a topic for assessment submission and in dissertations. Within the course content there was greater debate about the issues. The widening circles of communication within courses and within the project led to group sharing, discussions and enthusiasm as evidenced through the transcripts from the focus groups. Curriculum development has been enhanced through staff development and resources as the findings from PIPE activities were disseminated through the institutions. In one institution the delivery of the programme was restructured with enhanced focus on Illeris'[15] theoretical framework, explicitly concentrating on the group process. When the programmes are reviewed there will be more focus on modules dedicated to interprofessional learning.

Student satisfaction

The student evaluations of the modules and programmes gave positive feedback in relation to the enhanced focus on interprofessional learning. These were evidenced through verbal and written evaluations specifically related to shared and interprofessional and interdisciplinary learning and on discussing values and differences. There was also evidence of this in the student focus groups and questionnaires.

Another outcome is the dissemination by course students of PIPE activities in their work, this was demonstrated by student portfolios of evidence and assessment.

Curriculum changes: faculty and school level

While the focus on preparing for facilitation of interprofessional learning has been enhanced on teacher preparation programmes it is also an emergent theme in other new courses. For example, it is a burgeoning theme in new undergraduate nursing programmes currently being developed and implemented and this is enhanced by the dissemination of the PIPE project. Courses for practice teaching and mentorship also have an enhanced focus on facilitating interprofessional learning and interprofessional working.

Impact on faculties and schools

These have been far-reaching and have impacted on staff and in clinical practice. Qualitatively, there has been a dissemination of interest in IPL, formal and informal. This has had an impact on staff development, creating a change in culture with enhanced staff development and learning resources dedicated to IPL developments. It has provided an opportunity for university and clinical practice staff to undertake continuing professional development focused on interprofessional learning. Quantitatively, it has increased the number of staff and students, preparing to be teachers, with both knowledge and experience of IPL. It is to be expected that this will lead to a 'new breed' of educators/practitioners whose practice will continue to have influence.

Project level

Although it took some time for the initiative in PIPE scheme two to gather momentum and develop shared understanding, it has provided a forum for discussion among those managing these programmes for teacher preparation and led to changes in all of the programmes. Discussion and debate of the tensions in balancing the demands of education and practice were far-reaching. There was a comprehensive debate of the demands, philosophical and theoretical underpinnings and validity supporting the nature of these programmes as well as the most effective ways to approach preparing teachers to facilitate interprofessional learning. Postgraduate and post-registration programmes in healthcare were increasingly being developed as multidisciplinary, as well as featuring as a major theme in undergraduate programmes within the institutions. The transcripts from the students and programme teams did not allow distinction between the pre-existing conditions within the programmes, so it was not possible to say that one approach was better than another. Suggestions of approaches that enhance or hinder facilitation were the best that could be achieved.

The PIPE project provided a forum for discussion and dissemination of the PIPE research findings and activities from all of the elements of the project. It provided robust evidence that was lacking, to be disseminated to colleagues and students across the higher education institutions and in practice regarding the facilitation of interprofessional learning. The PIPE transferability period allowed attendance at local, professional, interprofessional, national and international conferences which has focused interest on the preparation of teachers and facilitators and on the vital role of the facilitator in interprofessional groups.

Usefulness of the sustainability framework

Each of the four higher education institutions prepared a summary document based on the sustainable interprofessional learning framework. Addressing the elements was useful in providing a clear focus for clarifying the changes that had been made within programmes and institutions. When these documents were integrated into the summary document (*see* Figure 6.2), they provided a very useful vehicle for comparison of similarities and differences. However the exact changes that have been made are difficult to capture.

Influences and motives for IPL in teacher preparation programmes

One major influence is the disparity in the educational preparation of teachers required by the health and social care professions. These range from the very specific requirements laid down by the Nursing and Midwifery Council for programmes at postgraduate diploma level to none. Although the four universities involved all required new lecturers to undertake programmes to meet the Higher Education Academy's standards for teachers, this does not apply to existing lecturers employed in higher education, or to those not on university contracts of employment. The four universities' programmes also had very different histories, as can be seen in the case studies above. Three had their origins in nursing and midwifery education, being guided primarily by their professional body regulations. Although they shared the common ground of meeting the Higher Education Academy's requirements for membership, their emphases were different, especially the emphasis on work-based, practice education in the three healthcare-based programmes. However, at the level of incorporating one common learning outcome these different backgrounds did not prove to be a barrier, but it would be a major factor if further curricular collaboration was envisaged. At present the programmes are only at the beginning of the evolution model stage. It is questionable if the revolutionary model of common curricular development needing formal inter-institutional contractual arrangements such as fee-for-service partnerships, collaborative partnerships or a consortium as described by Iwasiw *et al*[1] will be contemplated in the near future as the universities remain competitors. Being involved in PIPE enabled each to enhance their individual programmes, with no risk of losing business. Another educational influence on this initiative was the revisiting of curriculum models and frameworks. Interest in this field has been generated by the Higher Education Academy's imaginative curriculum project initiated by its previous generic centre network[16] and by authors such as Barnett and Coate.[17] This work sets the PIPE project in a context in which new approaches to curriculum development are being discussed and explored, providing an opening that interprofessional learning can exploit.

Conclusion: implications for curriculum development learned from the PIPE project

There are varying perspectives including different understandings of what constitutes knowledge and what are appropriate ways to approach teaching and learning in the health and social care professions. Courses have different cultures even within the same profession and therefore any attempt to define the curriculum may be contentious. One of the emerging issues from the PIPE project, was that one approach 'will not fit all'.

It was not possible to take one model of integrating the learning outcome and say it was better than another. The focus on interprofessional learning through PIPE has changed all the courses and all the programmes were enhanced, albeit differently, in each of the higher education institutions. A key aspect to be considered is that curriculum is a public or concrete statement of a process.[18] There should be an exploration and explanation of values and ideology, including a statement on position and the direction a course can be expected to take. Any constraints should be acknowledged and a rationale for selection of content and also for elements considered and rejected. Using Illeris'[15] Tension Triangle to reconcile conflicting demands for content and process has been successfully used in the PIPE project.

This knowledge is needed when producing curricula for whole programmes and on a smaller scale for modules or single sessions or study days. In health and social care education, several broad principles have been adopted which emphasise the following:

- promote learning and professionalism/professional relevance
- integrate theory with practice
- provide a person-centred approach to teaching and learning.

Outcomes from the PIPE project will influence curricula change, in particular the importance of the group development and the group learning process. Although no longer fashionable with the development of competence-based approaches, Stenhouse[18] advocates the process model and planning the curriculum as a totality and not in 'the piecemeal fashion hitherto adopted'. Lawton's ideal of selecting from the wider culture also has relevance in preparing and planning for interprofessional learning as this demands the participants to express the views and values that they perceive as important.[19]

Such areas that enhance interprofessional learning have been stated in the previous chapters and include developing a common language:

- awareness of and focus on group process
- some awareness of contact theory[20] and ethnocentrism[21]
- valuing the group members as individuals as well as professionals.

This last is echoed in the following statement from one programme team member:

> But I think for the students that one of the key things is that they start to see people – they see them as people – not just a midwife, a pharmacist. It's breaking down those barriers seems to be that social level which is very important. To treat people as people as opposed to their job label.

In developing curricula, certain key messages have emerged from the PIPE project. Curriculum development for single sessions or whole programmes is about developing learning opportunities for complex diverse collections of participants, and using Illeris[15] is a useful way of exploring the dimensions and tensions to provide balance. Gibson's work on the 'circumstantial curriculum' identifies that curricula should be situated in the complex world in which individuals practise with other practitioners.[22] Complexity is to be expected, but time invested in the group process will pay dividends: focusing on the barriers to learning in interprofessional settings helps to explore the topics of power and hierarchy as they exist in health and social care groups and teams. A strong recommendation has emerged, which is that time invested in developing the group is time well spent.

CHAPTER 7

Collaboration beyond champions

ANN EWENS AND GILL YOUNG

Introduction

The purpose of this chapter is to explore the role of champions, funding and inter-organisational partnerships in supporting interprofessional learning in the short and long term both in organisations and in practice.

There is a history within the higher education sector of short-term interprofessional learning projects that rarely make connections with core education programmes and tend to atrophy when funding ceases. To reduce the likelihood of this unfortunate outcome and to have a significant impact on practice, interprofessional learning needs to be established in all professional programmes at both pre- and post-registration levels. The challenge therefore, for sustainable interprofessional learning, is to move beyond short-term projects to establish sustainable programmes.

The question, 'can IPE be sustained within mainstream professional education once initial enthusiasm and earmarked funds run dry?'[1] posed in a recent position paper on interprofessional education in the UK, is what this chapter seeks to address. Mainstream in this context means operating as a core element within and across health and related organisations as opposed to the tenuous and marginal links that exist currently.

To enable an exploration of this key question related to establishing interprofessional learning within organisations where a short-term interprofessional project such as PIPE has been a catalyst; this chapter will focus on three aspects:

1 the role of champions
2 the impact of funding
3 inter-organisational partnerships.

The role of champions

Champions are individuals who have a major role in communicating and convincing others of their own beliefs and values in a particular area of interest such as interprofessional learning. Although they are often well-established, highly visible individuals who can lead change, they are, it is argued, unable to sustain programmes alone.[2] This view is supported by Freeth[3] where she identifies that interprofessional learning is dependent on key individuals, but that when they move on, or the project ends the initiatives they have championed and developed wither away.

Through exploring the characteristics of champions, it is possible to have an insight into their role in short-term interprofessional learning initiatives and understand what strategies they need to adopt to enable organisations to take these forward in the long term. Champions can be seen as people within organisations who have 'social and motivational qualifications'.[4] They have cooperation and communication abilities, initiative, drive and are able to keep up with, and contribute to developments. They are people who subscribe to a Foucaultian model of power, seeing it as existing only within social relationships, rather than the traditional model that sees power as a force held by a dominant group.[5] Champions understand the traditional hierarchical power dynamics and structures in their organisations, and can use this knowledge to make things happen, but do not personally subscribe to it. They view power as existing only within the immediate social relationship, whether it is an inter-organisational meeting or an inter-professional teaching session.

Champions are effective by putting themselves in a powerful position in their own organisation and in the partnership. They are able to wield influence within their organisation, not necessarily through their positional power, but by leading and influencing others, including those in positions of power into supporting a particular venture. They inspire others and lead by example towards a shared organisational goal. Champions have well-developed networks both within their organisation and in the wider world of health and social care which they use to bring about change.

It is these characteristics that define them as champions rather than as individuals who are totally committed to an idea, but who are limited in their ability to bring about change. An issue we have been asked about when presenting our work at conferences is, 'can you appoint someone to be an interprofessional learning champion?' The answer is yes. You need to identify someone in your organisation who is both passionate about interprofessional learning, and has the personal characteristics of a champion. When a project champion from one of the partner organisations leaves, it is important to replace that person with another champion. It is also imperative that if a major change such as this takes place within a project that the role of the person coming into a project is clearly outlined and efforts made to re-establish the team.

Champions play a pivotal role within a project such as PIPE, particularly in terms of inter-organisational partnership working in the short term. The champions have the ability to shape and sustain a project initially, but caution is needed if over-reliance is placed on expecting champions to be able to create new ways of working in their organisations in the long term. This is particularly so when working in a team, as partners within a project, where the members are all champions for interprofessional learning within their own organisations. It can lead to inter-dependence on each other for motivation but by fostering independence the project will move forward and be made sustainable in the long term. Consequently, to maximise the effectiveness of champions, strategies need to be adopted by them during the life of the project to work with the policies and infrastructures of their organisations and to begin to assist their organisations to establish interprofessional learning in their core educational programmes. Working in this way leads to knowledge development and enhances understanding of educational practices within the field. However, due to the champions' highly individualistic working style and beliefs, they also need to recognise the importance of an organisation's role in the long-term development of interprofessional learning. See Box 7.1 for recommended strategies. In addition, one of the challenges faced by this project and other Higher Education projects at the time, was that in seeking to gain wide representation onto the steering group, some of the people who were nominated as representatives did not necessarily have the personal commitment of a champion. This led to a failure to engage with the work of the project and had a potentially detrimental effect on the impact within those organisations. There are lessons to be learnt for funding bodies, who should monitor closely the continuing commitment of all who sign up to work together in a project.

BOX 7.1 Recommended strategies for long-term development

Champions need to create a formal mechanism to keep influential people in their organisations informed of developments to enable them to integrate developments into core programmes.

Champions need to start working with influential people in their own organisations, to create local policy and infrastructures for a long-term integration of the project aims and outcomes rather than wait until the end of the project.

Champions should highlight that their organisation needs to appoint others to take responsibility for taking the project outcomes forward in the long term. They need time to work alongside the champion before the project ends, and this could be between six and twelve months for long complex projects.

Impact of funding

As with most projects, the influence of the funding body is an important pressure on the parameters and direction of the initiative especially at the beginning and when the project is in its infancy. The prestige of having HEFCE funding provided a strong motivation for both the local champions and the organisations of PIPE as it helped the organisations involved to meet targets in a number of ways. Since these monies were for the development of teaching and learning in higher education, this motivated the partners to develop initiatives for investigation primarily in relation to teacher and facilitator preparation for interprofessional learning, rather than student learning.

An initiative such as the PIPE project is unlikely to develop without considerable monies, but funding can have a negative impact on sustainability, as partner organisations are unable or unwilling to provide continuity funding once the project monies end. At the end of the project there was an opportunity to continue some streams of work for a further six months with a bid for more funding (known as transferability funding). The requirement of the bid was that the funding was matched by the organisations involved. It was very encouraging that most of the partners agreed to provide and match the extra funding to continue the initiative for six more months. One of the questions the project team has had to address in evaluating this initiative is what prompted those organisations to commit more funding. The answer lies primarily in the fact that the project had been successful in involving key people from each of the organisations onto the steering group. They were able to commit funds on behalf of their organisations and thus express their personal commitment to interprofessional learning.

At this stage the project's ability to assist the organisations in achieving their objectives appeared to be a secondary consideration. Therefore, policies and infrastructure were not put in place to integrate interprofessional learning into the core educational programmes of all the institutions. This lack of integration was the reason why, at the end of the transferability-funding period, further funding was not forthcoming although the steering group members were keen to see the individual champions involved continue to work together. One of the challenges had been that the project was unsuccessful in making the link clear between interprofessional learning for teachers and the success of some of the organisations in implementing interprofessional learning in pre- and post-registration education.

There was variable action and participation from the individual champions and organisations which was converted into inconsistent experience and development, with some individuals and organisations gaining far more than others. The establishment of partnership working was utilised more within some of the institutions than others, with some displaying a reluctance to move very far away from their local professional customs and habits. This was particularly so with the medical education, despite the unstinting dedicated work of those champions involved with the project. In addition, those who gained the most financially were not necessarily those who experienced the majority of development and change. Therefore, although funding was vital to initiate the project, it was interesting that it was not the only factor that impacted on outcomes. There were also unplanned gains for several of the partner organisations. For example, one organisation gained by the provision of experts from partner institutions for its validation panels; others gained because partners provided lecturers for their programmes. All of these challenges are part of the nature of interprofessional collaboration and it is only by discussing and meeting these challenges that interprofessional education will become embedded in the culture of health and social care. The level of impact on staff development of those involved in the project is arguably the greatest and most sustainable outcome. This is both with the academic staff and those involved in practice education which then impacts on the quality of the learning experience for the student.

Another issue concerns those who fund interprofessional learning. Barr and Ross[1] assert that achieving mainstream interprofessional learning will involve a change in the culture of professional education, supported unequivocally by senior management and backed by core educational funding. For the PIPE project there was no scope for reviewing the current funding and policy mechanisms and combining budgets in order to persuade the participating organisations to collaborate on interprofessional learning. Ginsberg and Tregunno[7] offer a useful insight into the development of interprofessional learning through an examination of organisational change and the significant role played by formal leaders. Funded projects provide an opportunity to develop interprofessional learning in a comfortable, low risk and non-threatening context but the likely outputs as borne out by PIPE are that changes are minimal and only at the margins of the organisations' structures. To change how interprofessional learning is provided the government needs to combine the education funding for all professional groups in health and social care and only commission professional education that explicitly includes interprofessional learning.

Inter-organisational partnerships

Partnerships, as described in this chapter, are formal arrangements between and among organisations.[6] The range of partner organisations involved in the PIPE project may appear to have been carefully planned, but it was more a case of a gathering of individuals with an interest in interprofessional education. See Box 7.2 below.

BOX 7.2 Case study for PIPE partnership

The partnerships that became the PIPE project were a mix of personal relationships, networking and invitation. The project began with two individuals based within what became the lead university. They conceived the project in response to a tender for projects from the Fund for the Development of Teaching and Learning (FDTL) Phase 4. Applicants were encouraged to involve partner organisations in their project. Another organisation was invited to participate in the bid. Within a week, other potential partners had heard about the bid and requested a desire to become involved. A four-organisation partnership was established. They then invited three more organisations to broaden the geographical area and to span health and social care. The result was a seven-partner project.

The nature of the partnership was determined by local organisational and funding body factors. Inter-organisational projects often result from local networks, contacts and funding body demands rather than the needs of the project on which they plan to work. However, the consortium offered a unique opportunity to move beyond the commitment of individuals to institutional commitment and embed interprofessional learning beyond the life of this initiative. The steering group was seen as a significant vehicle by which the project would achieve its aims and had representation at senior level from a number of national organisations. In many ways this was successful and the steering group participated in the project's development in a number of ways, with each member bringing their expertise to the group and the discussion.

With so many partners the project's focus needed to be considered carefully so that everyone felt that it would serve their purpose. Each of those involved was deemed to be a champion for interprofessional learning in their organisation. Once all the partners had committed themselves, the structure of the PIPE project was created with four distinct but related schemes. The structure was complex and difficult, and perhaps not the best approach to developing interprofessional learning, because of the distinct and potentially separate nature of the schemes. There is much to learn here for other initiatives, with advice to keep a project as simple as possible in order to obtain the best outcomes for those involved. It was, however, very important at this early stage to get the commitment of the individual champions so that they in turn could obtain commitment from their organisations.

In order to sustain the interprofessional outcomes in the long term, the project team needed to integrate the four schemes. The working process of each of the schemes was in itself an example of interprofessional education and demonstrated the value of working together and how this in turn enabled learning together. The champions involved put a lot of energy and enterprise into establishing complex but functional networks from which new knowledge definitely emerged. However, the focus tended to be on the day-to-day workings of the project and it was not until the project's evaluation phase that attempts were made to bring the four schemes together. Two of the four schemes had complementary objectives, so their outcomes were closely integrated. However, the other two schemes were less integrated and encompassed the organisations who were more reluctant to change and therefore the overall structure and outcomes of the project were fragmented. This adversely affected the long-term integration of the project in the partner organisations and resulted in a reluctance by organisations to fund outcomes that did not meet their needs. The reality of inter-institutional collaboration is no less complex than that of interprofessional collaboration and there are many barriers that need to be overcome. There are a maze of complex and inter-related issues including discussion on what is meant by 'institution' and the implications for collaboration and the impact of differing priorities and motivation. It takes a willingness to question, challenge and change existing practice and the consideration of interprofessional learning as an imperative versus an optional extra.

The lessons to take from this are that when organisations form a partnership it is often initially in response to interest from their local champions. Ultimately, this only leads to sustained interest and commitment when it benefits the organisation in reaching its objectives. On looking back at the project and the behaviour of the partners, it is now possible to see a complex mixture of socially-orientated values regarding the promotion of interprofessional learning for the common good, alongside the more commercial motivations of organisations that were competing for students. The visible signs of commitment by the partners are included in Box 7.3.

BOX 7.3 Commitment by partners

- Willingness to explore each other's curricula.
- Willingness to change and reorganise teaching timetables to allow for interprofessional events to take place.
- Willingness to provide staff time off beyond that funded by the project.
- Willingness to provide venues and facilities.
- Willingness to commit funds to extend the project.

These visible signs of commitment are important. Challenging this overt support for interprofessional learning across the partner institutions, the views expressed by Ginsburg and Tregunno[7] need to be considered. They posited that organisations are willing to respond to mild changes in the way they operate, for example, in terms of interprofessional learning providing that it does not involve a fundamental change to the 'deep structure' of the organisation. They further claim that major changes within organisations are very difficult, and only threats of organisational failure provide the impetus for change.

In considering the PIPE project, in terms of the organisational commitment of its partners, there was no challenge at any time to any of the partners to respond by making major changes to the working of their organisations. Looking at the partnerships involved in the project, it would be highly unlikely that the project could have influenced any of the partner organisations to engage in a major change towards how interprofessional learning was conducted. For example, one of the project schemes aimed to look at teacher training programmes across four of the seven partner organisations. Although a common learning outcome was successfully introduced into all the postgraduate teacher and facilitator preparation programmes and the work of the project actually informed and changed parts of the curriculum, they were unable to create a common module as initially planned. This would have required a greater commitment, and curriculum review and revalidation to make this more radical change.

Ginsburg and Tregunno[7] state that whilst 'change champions' can have a significant impact upon interprofessional learning, it is essential that formal leaders provide the necessary support for organisational change. Formal leaders, they claim, set the strategic direction for change, establish the structure and parameters for implementation, allocate resources and stimulate the interest and commitment of others in the organisation. Through reviewing the literature, they identified that evidence exists to support the idea of leader commitment and ongoing involvement as a key feature of successful long-term organisational change.

Through analysis of 'institutional theory' Ginsburg and Tregunno[7] also noted that the external environment has a significant impact upon organisations, with outside pressure leading to uniformity across organisations. They claim that an effective way of bringing about change is to use coercive measures through regulatory bodies or by change at policy level. This idea links to their earlier point about how organisations tend only to make major changes when the future of the organisation is under threat.

Whilst external policies and professional bodies explicitly promote interprofessional learning and support interprofessional initiatives, the discipline specific funding for education does not encourage interprofessional learning. For example, funding is provided for uni-disciplinary education in health and social care in England not interdisciplinary education. In exploring the Canadian context of funding for healthcare education, Gilbert[8] identified the impact of external agencies and professional bodies on universities, and stated that funding is discipline-bound and that when funding is cut, it is usually education that is not uni-disciplinary that suffers. He also identified that university structures do not encourage cross faculty developments, and that there are no established funding models to promote this.

These concerns about establishing interprofessional learning are also reflected in the views of lecturers in the partner organisations who were involved in interprofessional learning in the classroom. In research undertaken as part of the project, lecturers on the programme teams, and student teachers on the teacher and facilitator preparation programmes in four of the partner institutions were interviewed. Below are two of the key items that emerged from the data.

1 Hierarchical structures within and between the NHS, social care and the higher education sector, are perceived as barriers to interprofessional learning and working. This is particularly the case with the older universities where the majority of medical and dental education has traditionally taken place.

2 The development of interprofessional learning tends to be context-specific, dependent primarily on individuals' commitment rather than being embedded at professional or organisational level.

In summary, organisational commitment to a particular project or initiative will be demonstrated by the provision of resources and strategies to support change. However, these are more often seen in situations where organisations engage in low risk minor changes that do not challenge the deep structures of the organisation in question. There is also a recognition that funding and resource restriction has the potential to inhibit the extent to which change can be embedded because of the finite timescale of a project. Organisations are only likely to engage in major changes when under threat. This also extends to the practice environment, where permanent change is dependent on practice-based staff changing their practice or expectations, which may be even harder to achieve in the work environment. If interprofessional learning is to become a core activity, the regulatory bodies, senior management and funding bodies must be wholly committed to it. The strategies in Box 7.4 demonstrate to organisations how to make long-term changes in their operation.

BOX 7.4 Strategies to engage organisations

- Initially identify and gain commitment from champions who can 'kick start' an initiative and establish links with those who have power and influence.
- Include those who hold influential power in the structure of the project, i.e. steering group. This allows the project team to capitalise on their socially-orientated values towards the project goals.
- Establish as early as possible how the structure and outcomes of the project will integrate long-term into the core business of the partner organisations.
- Be willing to adapt the structure and outcomes of the project to achieve long-term sustainability and implementation of its main aims.
- Assess the likely impact and ability of the project to influence the policy and infrastructure of partner organisations through activities external to the partnerships.
- Following the above assessment accept the scope of the project, and work towards achievable goals.

Conclusion

This chapter has explored the issue of establishing interprofessional learning beyond short-term projects and beyond the champions. It has identified a number of issues that need to be taken into consideration when setting up a similar venture to that of the PIPE project. Firstly, that whilst champions are vital in getting an initiative off the ground, losing a champion can have a damaging impact on the outcomes of an initiative. It is essential that formal support and organisational commitment, for the right reasons, is achieved in order to gain long-term change to the core business of partner organisations. Formal support is most likely to be accomplished if the project is designed from the beginning to integrate interprofessional learning with the policies and infrastructure of the organisations involved. However, the quantitative understanding of the perceived impact of a project such as PIPE is impossible to establish in a simple cause and effect relationship. In today's world of evidence-based practice, measuring the impact is an inevitably imprecise process. Perhaps the most significant impact is on the development of the people themselves who are involved with a project and is arguably the most sustainable impact. Since this in turn creates and develops individual champions who have the personal commitment and drive to take the belief forward wherever they are and for whichever organisation they work for.

Interprofessional learning initiatives such as the PIPE project can provide incentives for organisations to work at establishing interprofessional learning, providing the project does not challenge their stability. If major change is desired, then a short-term project can only be part of the strategy, as greater incentives will be needed to encourage organisations to take risks in order to sustain such work. It is suggested that these champions themselves, will ultimately be the ones in a position to establish interprofessional learning beyond the life of the project they were involved with.

CHAPTER 8

Through the PIPE

ELIZABETH HOWKINS AND JULIA BRAY

Introduction

In this final chapter, the learning and evidence from the PIPE project presented in the previous chapters will be drawn together to address the question:

> What needs to be in place to develop, sustain and embed the preparation of facilitators of IPL for health and social care, both in the formal education setting and in practice?

Many aspects concerning the development of facilitators for IPL, the curriculum, the theories, the practice and the inter-institutional collaboration have already been discussed and some frameworks and action points presented to take forward. But how to develop, sustain and embed quality facilitation for IPL is more challenging. We have not found a panacea on which to base all facilitator preparation, and proposing only one way would be restrictive, but we have devised a set of principles for it. In understanding the facilitator role for IPL, we realised that nothing should be implemented in practice without acknowledging the impact of the wider political, organisational and professional context in which it takes place. In order to set our work in context we will set out a strategy for IPL facilitator preparation.

The chapter covers four areas, with the first two providing a brief reminder of why IPL facilitation needs improving and where it takes place. The third area will examine the lessons learnt from the PIPE project using the emerging evidence and present a set of principles for IPL facilitation. The fourth area will propose an IPL facilitation preparation strategy.

The need to improve IPL facilitation

During the PIPE project it became clear that despite over a decade of work by the UK government on improving interprofessional education within health and social care, much still remains to be done. Interprofessional education is now being incorporated into the mainstream of professional education for health and social care professionals throughout the UK. 'Mainstreaming interprofessional education' as it is referred to, aims to integrate IPE into organisational, financial and theoretical terms for professional education.[1] An example of the UK government's commitment to mainstreaming interprofessional education can be found in the Department of Health funded project; 'Creating an Interprofessional Workforce Programme (CIPW)'[2] which aims to produce an education and training framework for health and social care in England.

However, in order to sustain interprofessional working, there needs to be an effective balance between the provision of IPL in higher education and the opportunities in practice. Effective IPL needs support at many levels, as professionals working in practice are likely to become disillusioned if their efforts to work collaboratively are not effective. This is particularly so for those students emerging from ambitious pre-qualifying programmes, incorporating interprofessional working, into a workforce where the reality of collaborative working is very different. Ross and Barr[3] refer to the thrust in identifying how interprofessional learning can continue in the workplace and the need to focus attention on ways in which learning occurs, or fails to occur.

The importance of staff development to improve facilitation on interprofessional education programmes is now well documented.[4,5] Throughout the PIPE project, the assumption was that by improving IPL facilitation the experience of IPL will improve, which in turn will improve patient/client care. Evidence has already been discussed in earlier chapters that poor facilitation can have a negative effect on the outcomes of any IPL session. However, in the workplace, there is a paradox. IPL sessions are set up as multiprofessional, to address a shared area of work (for example: the introduction of the Single Assessment Process (SAP) as part of the National Service Frameworks for older people).[6] But the emphasis is often on giving information with the process of learning to work collaboratively frequently ignored. The assumption, that by putting professionals together to learn, they will then work together, is a flawed assumption. The lack of preparation given to the group facilitator and the expectation that, because someone is an experienced practitioner, they will effectively manage interprofessional and inter-agency group learning, is misguided. We would argue from the evidence that we found in PIPE, that health and social care organisations are wasting valuable resources by organising interprofessional sessions in the workplace run by inadequately prepared facilitators.

The need, therefore, to improve the quality of IPL facilitation is compelling, both in the workplace and in higher education.

Places where IPL facilitation takes place

Throughout this book we have demonstrated that facilitation of IPL takes place in many different settings. Some in formal education settings, many work-based educational sessions and a very large number of opportunistic activities where an interprofessional learning situation occurs which, with skilled handling, could be turned into an effective learning opportunity in the practice setting. During the final stages of the project transferability period, as part of the dissemination strategy, we ran workshops both in higher education institutions and in practice. One of the main unanticipated outcomes was the tremendous response from practice to the workshops. We ran six workshops which were all attended by professionals from a range of diverse backgrounds. We were surprised at how many very senior staff attended, including a number of doctors. The sessions provided some important learning for us as a team and identified some particular examples of learning opportunities. The following real scenario (Box 8.1) sets out this potential IPL opportunity.

BOX 8.1 The PIPE workshop for facilitation of IPL in the workplace

The workshops had been advertised widely through the Health Trust training calendar and the response was very pleasing with a diverse range of professionals attending. This included general practitioners, public health nurses, consultants, as well as workers from other areas such as Teenage Pregnancy and Sure Start projects.

In setting up the programme we intended to model the teaching methods and styles we would be recommending for those facilitating groups in practice to ensure that interactive learning took place. We also included work on group dynamics and adult learning, as well as ways of sustaining and developing IPL.

In the evaluation of the first session there was some feedback that the information on IPL was not relevant to those attending and, although the day had been successful, we were aware that some parts of the session were not well received and the group had 'switched off'!

After rigorously going through the evaluations, we sat down and looked again at the programme before the next session and revised it. We made the decision to take out the overt references to IPL but to make the interprofessional learning elements of the day more implicit. The next session was again well attended and, at an appropriate point, we asked who, in the group of 20, was involved in IPL. Only one person replied that they were. We then found out which of them worked in teams, who ran sessions for other professionals and who taught other professionals as part of their work, etc. This lead to a discussion on IPL. Although they were all involved in IPL, they had not realised it. This was a revelation to us and would be an interesting subject to research further. If professionals do not think they are facilitating IPL groups, they will not be interested in the research, advice and support that is available on IPE.

We continued with this format and the sessions were very lively, interesting and very well evaluated.

We took a valuable lesson from this sobering experience which highlighted that teaching on facilitation of IPL must be accessible at many different levels. This includes professionals with some formal preparation of teaching, practice educators and expert practitioners with facilitation experience. However, for us it identified the biggest challenge as the need to reach practitioners who may not realise that they have a significant role to play in promoting IPL. Preparation for becoming a facilitator should be available to any practitioner and acknowledged as part of their continuing professional development (CPD) if they are facilitating interprofessional groups.

In the next section we used the lessons from PIPE to set out a framework to guide the development of facilitator preparation.

Lessons learnt from the PIPE project

The problem that the PIPE team grappled with was whether there really was something extra about teaching/facilitating interprofessional learning and, if so, what was it? At the start of the project we probably anticipated that we would develop a set of skills, some teaching tools, some knowledge and, we hoped, some theory to guide the process of facilitator preparation for IPL. We did, in fact, learn some very useful approaches to teaching; we identified some characteristics essential to facilitation and we proposed a theoretical framework that should help programme planners and curriculum developers for IPL. But overall, what we found was that effective IPL facilitation requires more than skills and knowledge; it requires a set of values which have to become a way of life for the facilitator and their organisation. We have incorporated these into a set of principles for the IPL facilitator based on our research and evaluation which has been fully discussed throughout the book.

Principles for an IPL facilitator
- A commitment to collaborative learning.
- A commitment to the learner as the most important learning resource for IPL.
- Acknowledging and using other's professional experience.
- Using and working with professional power.
- Respecting and welcoming difference in all people and professions.
- Expecting, engaging with, and learning from tension and conflict.
- Using and developing reflection.
- Making professional jargon explicit in the group.
- Investing time in the pre-planning with all stakeholders.
- Investing time in group development.
- Knowing and understanding self in role.
- Awareness of own behaviour in modelling IPL.

The above set of principles present a rather daunting list and it is important to establish how this relates to the provision of IPL teaching in the workplace and higher education. It also raises the question of how preparation for this facilitator role really can be made accessible to more practitioners? The CIPW strategy[2] is based on evidence that being interprofessional enhances profession specific identity and, certainly with the changing landscape facing the provision of health and social care in the UK today and in the future, the need to be interprofessional becomes a necessary attribute for all professionals. Throughout the project, we collected a lot of information and evidence about the types of IPL taking place, and to start this discussion it is helpful to outline the characteristics that are recognised in shaping IPL in the workplace.

Characteristics that shape IPL in the workplace

- Workforce learning is based on real life and should reflect organisational need.
- Professionals come to IPL sessions strongly influenced by their own professional beliefs and values.
- Opportunities which offer potential for IPL should be used wherever possible.
- Organisations need to prepare and support facilitators to promote IPL in the workplace.
- Within organisations there needs to be shared understanding of the meaning of IPL.

These are all characteristics that many organisations may feel they already accept and are working towards, based on excellent teamwork, good communication and an understanding of professional roles. However, these are difficult and demanding areas of human relationships which should be part of every organisation's continuing professional development programme. The health and social care organisations are; education providers, in-service training, health and social care employers, practitioners, voluntary services, professional bodies and education policy makers. It is therefore fundamental to work with these organisations to set out a shared framework which takes in to account the wider political and organisational context in which IPL facilitation takes place. Ultimately to take forward the work of the PIPE project and embed quality IPL facilitation across both higher education and in the workplace requires a sound realistic strategy.

IPL facilitation preparation strategy

Drawing on the evidence from the PIPE project, three areas that make up a proposed IPL preparation facilitation strategy will be discussed and explored. These are:

1 the importance of staff development and facilitator preparation for IPL
2 curriculum development for IPL facilitation
3 educational funding and policy to support for IPL.

The importance of staff development and facilitator preparation for IPL

The results of our research about the development of IPL facilitator skills and knowledge showed that the facilitator role was demanding and required a high level of expertise to facilitate IPL groups, which are, by their nature diverse and complex. We identified five main categories to guide a facilitator in their preparation and in the process of the group facilitation. They are:

1 awareness and use of self as a facilitator
2 dealing with difference and conflict
3 group process and relationships
4 power dimensions for facilitator and group
5 context and planning.

The above have been discussed at length in Chapter 3 and other chapters in the book so will not be repeated here. Our challenge now is to accept that training in facilitation should be available to all practitioners in the following ways:

■ formal facilitator preparation courses run in higher education
■ facilitator preparation supporting multiprofessional qualifying courses in HEI
■ in-service day courses
■ study days in the work base
■ action learning sets in practice
■ buddy scheme set up to receive feedback on facilitation
■ personal development plan supported by experienced facilitator.

Many of these approaches have been raised in previous chapters of this book with the formal education courses detailed in Chapter 4 and the work based initiatives in Chapter 5. None of the approaches set out should be seen as the best, or only way to learn facilitation of IPL. The complexity of the role and the length of time needed to gain experience means practitioners undertaking any level of IPL facilitation role should have some form of preparation. The lack of awareness that interprofessional work and learning is part of the role of all practitioners requires a culture shift that must take place. Thus, by incorporating the facilitation role into staff development to make it part of the professional development programme could help change attitudes as people learn new skills and become more aware of their role in opportunistic IPL facilitation. Supporting practitioners in their new roles as facilitators must be ongoing with time given to reflect on facilitation experiences and opportunities to co-facilitate with an experienced facilitator. In this way, facilitator preparation would slowly become embedded in interprofessional practice.

Curriculum development for IPL facilitation

The curriculum is central to the planning of interprofessional learning sessions.

The learners in any interprofessional group are a diverse complex collection of people who require learning opportunities tailored to their needs, so that they are enabled to learn 'with, from and about' each other. These demands are the same even if it is for one study day, several study days or a whole teacher preparation programme. In addition any courses for IPL, whether long, short or single days should demonstrate that they are based on an integrated IPL curriculum. The interprofessional aspect for any programme must not just appear as, 'an add on', to the main content but be part of a well thought out plan.

It was the results of the research undertaken by scheme two in the PIPE project that further illuminated the approach for IPL preparation. The group started by addressing the issue of the increasing focus on interprofessional learning for teacher preparation programmes at masters level. The challenge to the group was how to incorporate IPL into teacher preparation programmes and the broad research question was:

> How can IPL most effectively be incorporated into postgraduate teaching programmes?

The results of the study provided three themes for how essential characteristics for IPL facilitation might be developed among healthcare professionals involved as students or as programme team members on education programmes for health and social care professionals. These themes are:

1 experiencing IPL as an approach to professional practice
2 experiencing modelling of IPL in a variety of contexts, both educational and practice based
3 opportunities to reflect on the challenges of IPL.

These three themes provide a secure framework within which those developing their skills as educators can develop their understanding of IPL and begin the process of making informed choices.

A strategic aim for all IPL facilitator preparation should be to have quality courses, both in formal education and in the workplace. To achieve these aims curricula should embrace the approaches and values outlined in the three themes framework and ensure that interprofessional learning outcomes are always fully integrated within any IPL facilitation programme.

Educational funding for and policy to support IPL

The opportunity offered through the PIPE project for a collaborative project was quite special and unusual. The partners to the project consisted of five HEIs with two other partners, the Oxford Deanery and Social Work training development agency (the latter left the project after the first year). The steering group was made up of senior members from all these organisations, which for them offered a unique opportunity to explore a subject that would no doubt have been very low on their agenda. In addition, it is interesting to note that all the HEIs are in competition with each other for their student cohorts, so they would not normally have risked sharing initiatives about individual programmes. However the interest and depth of discussion at the steering group meetings and the progress made was considerable and consistent. An example of the depth of support for the project from the steering group was shown in their willingness to individually fund the transferability period of six months. At the end of this period efforts were made to get some ongoing work in place and a limited agreement was made, but it was clear that once the funding ceased the input into collaborative work on IPL would eventually end.

The lessons learnt from the collaborative aspect of the project can no doubt be reflected in many other funded projects. The level of collaboration, the scale of work, and the activities of the champions drive the project during its life, but do not continue without educational policy and ring fenced money.

The activities of 'mainstreaming interprofessional education'[3] and hopefully the outcomes of the Department of Health project 'Creating an interprofessional workforce programme'[2] should have some impact on ways to make interprofessional education and the preparation of facilitators for IPL become educational policy with money to support the policy.

We do recommend the findings of our PIPE project as strong evidence that money spent on quality IPL facilitation preparation at all levels of professional development makes sound economic sense and should be part of any staff development budget.

Conclusion

The PIPE project aim was to find ways to improve teacher/facilitator preparation for IPL, in both academic settings and in the workplace to ensure high quality teaching of IPL. In the book we have set out our learning in the form of research-based evidence, some frameworks, possible theories and ideas, practical suggestions and a set of principles for the role of IPL facilitator. This final chapter offered an overview of the project findings and a number of proposals on how to develop, sustain and embed the preparation of facilitators of IPL for health and social care.

The development of facilitators can be guided by the set of principles for IPL facilitation, either as an approach to facilitation and/or to underpin any preparation course. In addition the three themes framework will help educators to understand the IPL process and make informed choices within any programme development.

Sustaining IPL facilitation preparation is demanding and it needs a shift in attitude by all potential partners to accept that it is not just for an elite group, but for a large number of practitioners. PIPE should not be seen as only for academics, it is about linking the workplace and academia to improve the quality of facilitation for IPL. The greatest promise for promoting interprofessional learning is a synergy between the workplace and academic domains.

Embedding facilitation for IPL could be achieved through a government funded strategy that involves all the potential partner organisations to put in place a workable and quality framework which promotes the preparation of facilitators for IPL in health and social care.

As a project team we are now at the end of our journey, we have come 'through the PIPE', learnt that it is a complex and difficult journey, full of new pipes, dead end pipes, pipes that join us to others, reservoir pipes, and final pipes leading to some solution. Our PIPE metaphor has been useful in realising that complexity and uncertainty are an integral part of a large research evaluation study. The process of trying to make sense of the data, producing some wise words and having a practical application have been huge challenges. But we have been able to draw conclusions from our material to produce a set of principles for the

IPL facilitator and an IPL facilitation preparation strategy. We held a conference at the end of the project and the theme was 'More than just a PIPE dream' as IPL is not just a dream and not just a project but a reality in today's world. The conference was seen as an excellent opportunity to not only celebrate and share the work of the PIPE project but to openly celebrate the diversity, innovation and excellence widely evident in the field of interprofessional education both nationally and internationally. Finally, our PIPE journey can be summed up in words spoken by Sir Winston Churchill:

Out of intense complexities, intense simplicities emerge.

The PIPE project

ELIZABETH HOWKINS AND JULIA BRAY

The idea became reality through a chance meeting in a corridor between two champions of interprofessional education. Together they tapped into their networks of local people interested in improving teaching interprofessional education, both in practice and in higher education. It was also at an opportunistic time, as some informal collaborative work was already underway between two of the eventual PIPE education partners. The eventual success in getting government funding gave a group of doctors, nurses, social workers and allied health professionals from the Thames Valley area, the valuable time to share and explore the many issues associated with promoting and facilitating interprofessional education.

The strength of the PIPE project team was the wealth of knowledge they bought with them, both as professionals and educationalists. In the early days there were many aspects related to teaching interprofessional education that the group debated and discussed, but the main underlying issue was that practitioners and teachers often felt ill prepared for facilitating interprofessional learning both in higher education and in practice. The problem that the team grappled with, was the need to discover whether there really was something additional or extra about teaching IPE and, if there was, what was it?

The term **interprofessional learning** will be used in the next section as in the rest of the book. It was the term constantly used by the project team throughout the life of the project. A fuller discussion on the usage of the terms, interprofessional education and interprofessional learning can be found in Chapter 1, Section one.

The PIPE project

The bid for the PIPE project was submitted to the Higher Education funding council in May 2002 following discussions between numbers of professionals in the Thames Valley area involved in interprofessional education. The opportunity for funding arose from the UK's Higher Education Funding Council's phase four grant for the development of teaching and learning in Higher Education Institutions (Funding for the Development of Teaching and Learning FDTL4). This led to a consortium of organisations consisting of five Higher Education Institutions, University of Reading (host institution), Buckinghamshire Chiltern

University College, Oxford University, Oxford Brookes University and Thames Valley University as well as the Oxford Deanery for Postgraduate Dental and Medical Education. The grant was for three years to develop the facilitators/educators/teachers of interprofessional learning (IPL) across these organisations and was followed by a further successful bid (transferability) for eight months to disseminate the outcomes of the project further. The focus emerged from the original discussions on concerns around the preparation of teachers/facilitators to teach IPL and is the theme throughout the book. The project commenced in January 2003 and completed in 2007, with the outcomes and evaluation of the project now making an important contribution to the emerging evidence base on facilitation of interprofessional learning.

The structure of the PIPE project emerged from the need to allow for the many facets of IPL in health and social care to be addressed (see project scheme outline below). The professionals responsible for the bid were all champions of IPL involved with the preparation of professionals for teaching but representing many different areas. This covered a wide range including undergraduate medical students at Oxford University, undergraduate nursing and allied health professionals at two of the universities, lecturers in higher education and practice educators and general practitioners (GPs) on preparation courses as educators of GPs.

The aims of the PIPE project:

- to develop the preparation of teaching staff for interprofessional learning (IPL) across health and social care
- to develop effective strategies for collaboration between project partners
- to disseminate the findings from the project across health, social care and higher education.

To meet these needs the project structure involved four distinct but related schemes across six organisations, each with a scheme leader and working towards a joint set of objectives, seeking to ensure high quality teaching. In essence, the PIPE team were striving for continuous quality improvement in IPL at undergraduate and postgraduate level, through the educational institutions and in the workplace by improved teacher/facilitator preparation. The project was directed and led by a project director and the project team comprised of four scheme leaders and representatives from each of the organisations involved.

PIPE scheme one

The focus of this scheme was to develop and evaluate the transition of the established New Trainers Course in Oxford Postgraduate Deanery from a medically led course for doctors to an interprofessional course for all primary healthcare professionals.

The project team was made up of members of staff from Oxford Postgraduate Medical Education Deanery and Oxford Brookes University.

PIPE scheme two

The aims of scheme two were to enhance the focus on interprofessional learning in each of the postgraduate programmes in professional education and to develop evidence-based guidelines for the incorporation of IPL into such programmes elsewhere.

The partners were Oxford Brookes University, Buckinghamshire Chilterns University College, Reading University and Thames Valley University.

PIPE scheme three

The aim of scheme three was to explore the development of the skills and teaching methods needed for the preparation of facilitators undertaking IPL in the work base.

The scheme team comprised of the scheme leader from University of Reading, the project lead and representatives from the other higher education institutions.

PIPE scheme four

The main objective of scheme four was to prepare facilitators for developing inter-professional learning in undergraduate education. The remit was to focus on those teaching undergraduate and pre-qualifying health and social care students. This scheme took a realistic approach in focusing on only two of the higher education institutions within the consortium (Oxford University and Oxford Brookes University) although the lessons were likely to be transferable across the other higher education institutions, within and beyond this consortium.

Within the project as a whole, as an inter-organisational collaboration, the steering group was seen as a significant vehicle by which the project would achieve its aims and had representation at senior level from all the six organisations. In addition, the steering group had representation from the Thames Valley Workforce Development Confederation, the Higher Education Academy subject centre for Health Sciences and Practice and CAIPE (Centre for Advancement for Interprofessional Education). The steering group was ably chaired by Professor Gibson who is the Director of Teaching and Learning from the University of Reading BUILT Environment. The input from this completely different profession brought with it interesting perspectives, as the problems they have in developing collaborative working mirror the challenges faced in health and social care.

At the outset of the project there was representation from social work with the Training and Service Development agency for social care represented on the project team and steering group. However, quite soon this organisation dissolved and the team were left with a problem on how to meet this shortfall. A large amount of time was expended by the project lead and the scheme leaders to replace the social care element but without success. The team eventually came to the conclusion that it was not going to be possible to find representation at steering group level but aimed to address the social care perspectives in other ways by having social workers on the scheme teams.

Representation at senior level from all of the organisations was seen as a useful indicator of the level of commitment within each organisation and in this respect, had varied success which is discussed in Chapter 7. However, the steering group participated in the project's development in a number of ways, with each member bringing their expertise and contacts to the discussion on the project process and outcomes. The team believed that the consortium offered a unique opportunity to move beyond the commitment of individuals to institutional commitment and embed interprofessional learning beyond the life of this specific initiative. The project also had a student panel, representing the 'user input' from the organisations involved and had representation on the steering group.

The project has been instrumental in stimulating dialogue between all of these organisations and local, regional and national groups. It has acted as a catalyst to bringing people and organisations together in a variety of ways and this is highlighted throughout the book. The project team have worked together to disseminate the work both at national and international levels with presentations, workshops and participation at conferences. This has been very effective at initiating and maintaining critical dialogue with professionals seeking to develop interprofessional learning in other settings.

Evaluation strategy of the PIPE project

It was decided at the beginning of the project that the evaluation would be fully integrated into the project's action plan and the responsibility of all participants in the project. At the commencement of the project an external evaluator and internal evaluator were appointed.

The evaluation was conducted at three levels:
1 evaluation of the project's progress and processes in relation to the aims and objectives of the project and to assess the effectiveness of the processes and procedures employed by the project team
2 evaluation of the project's deliverables and their impact
3 an external evaluator who monitored the evaluation strategy and advised at critical stages on all matters to do with the evaluation of the project.

An evaluation strategy was prepared which included an attitudinal survey of both students and staff. However, this questionnaire did not have a good response and was decided not to be a viable method of evaluating the work. There were also many changes in the project team at this point and the internal evaluator moved to another area. Consequently, the initial plans for evaluation changed and the strategy was re-appraised. At that point it was decided that the project team would carry out the internal evaluation, whilst the external evaluator would remain to provide an overview of the success of the project and advise when needed. We were fortunate enough to have the expertise of Dr Marilyn Hammick for the length of the project and some of the comments from her final report are quoted at the end of this section.

The strategy for internal evaluation had to take in to account the PIPE resources available. Two of the PIPE schemes (two and three) had planned to set up and undertake a research evaluation approach to their work which would demand much time and use of the already limited PIPE resources. In light of this, a decision regarding the overall PIPE evaluation was made to use the information produced from the four schemes' quarterly reports, the PIPE annual reports, the workshops, minutes of meetings, and conference dissemination. In addition 'three minute papers' were carried out at the end of the project meetings and scheme meetings requiring a three minute period where all of the participants in the meeting recorded whatever thoughts they wanted on a piece of paper. This data has provided valuable evidence on the ability to openly acknowledge and challenge our own and each other's perceptions and assumptions about education and practice.

All the evaluation material was systematically gathered throughout the life of the project, it was then interpreted, judgements made and recommendations formed the project outcomes.

In addition to the overall project evaluation, schemes two and three designed and undertook two rigorous research projects which are fully described in Chapters 3, 4 and 6 in the book, but a very brief overview is offered here.

Scheme two started by setting out a broad research question: how can IPL most effectively be incorporated into postgraduate teaching programmes? They then carried out an extensive series of focus groups undertaken with students from four Higher Education Institution (HEI) and programmed team members from each HEI. These were analysed using the Radnor (2001) framework[1] for interpretive analysis of qualitative educational data to identify themes associated with the incorporation of IPL into postgraduate programmes.

Scheme three's aim was to explore the development of the skills and teaching methods needed for the preparation of facilitators undertaking IPL in the work base. This was a very different focus from the other schemes which were all based on programmes in educational establishments. Scheme three team was led by a team leader from the University of Reading and consisted of members from each of the higher education institutions and the project lead. The challenge to PIPE three was to find out if there are additional skills and knowledge needed for facilitation of interprofessional learning in the workplace. A Delphi research study was designed to explore the facilitation skills and knowledge needed to promote effective IPL in the workplace.

The similar results from both the schemes provided validity and reliability to the whole project evaluation. The results from both the studies were used to strengthen the evidence for change in all of the other educational programmes throughout the project.

In the final external evaluation report Dr Marilyn Hammick commented that, 'the PIPE project had shown that, given a common factor (in this case, the political imperative of interprofessional education for under- and postgraduate health and social care learners) it is possible for multiple higher education institutions (HEI) to collaborate'. The following extracts are taken from the final evaluation report[2] by Dr Hammick:

... the project had demonstrated that working in this way leads to knowledge development and enhances understanding of educational practices in a given field, whilst an emergent and potential outcome of the project is the sustainability of complex networking structures once the original project is complete.

The working process of each PIPE scheme has been, in and of itself, an example of interprofessional education and the value of reflective practice by education practitioners. The development, delivery, and enquiries into the education interventions provided by the schemes demonstrate the value of working together and how this, in turn, enables learning together. The staff are to be congratulated for the effort, energy and enterprise they put into establishing complex but functional networks from which new knowledge most definitely emerged. The enquiry work was conducted in a sound, ethical and pragmatic manner and has contributed to the evidence base in the field. The working processes and outcomes are examples of best practice that are not only of value to the interprofessional health and social care education and practice community, nationally and internationally, but have a transferability to other collaborative ventures.

The simultaneous occurrence of the different processes has provided the evaluation with both scope and depth, greatly helping to assist the understanding of facilitation of IPL and how to prepare facilitators/teachers. The data has also provided fascinating material for ongoing scholarly activity that will be used in future publications and discussion that will continue beyond the end of the project.

PIPE three research methodology and methods

JULIA BRAY

Following the outlining of the framework in Chapter 3 and initial discussions with the project team, three questions emerged and were echoed throughout the work of the project:

- are the facilitation skills and knowledge necessary for facilitators of work-based interprofessional learning any different from the skills needed for facilitation of any other work-based group?
- if so how should they be promoted?
- and crucially, how are they to be acquired?

A literature review was carried out and the following research question was posed:

> What, if any, are the facilitation skills and knowledge needed to promote effective interprofessional learning in the workplace?

The research method utilised the Delphi technique which takes its name from the Delphic oracle of Ancient Greece, employing the skills of interpretation and foresight. It is a consensus method, synthesising a wide range of information in areas where there is little or no research. It seeks to overcome some of the disadvantages found in the decision making process and, according to Crotty,[1] is deemed an effective method for structuring group communication when dealing with a complex problem with the aim of gathering opinions and informing debate. The Delphi technique was thus selected to ascertain 'expert opinion' on the complexities of facilitating IPL where logistically it would have been difficult to bring participants together from a range of professionals in health and social care. The professional background of the respondents listed eight from a nursing background, five with a medical background, three allied health professionals, one teacher, and one National Health Service manager. It was unfortunate that despite approaching a number of representatives from social care we had no response from them in the survey.

The research process was initiated using a questionnaire produced online for the participants with the purpose of ascertaining quantitative information on professional background, training, etc. The questionnaire used in the second round was structured according to the feedback and results from the first round with the principal aim of establishing consensus on the knowledge and skills necessary for the facilitation of interprofessional learning.

Following the analysis of the second questionnaire, the final outcomes of the results demonstrated that to prepare facilitators for IPL they need to acquire advanced and in-depth skills of facilitation, similar to those required to facilitate other complex diverse groups. But more importantly the results produced some very rich data about the sort of skills, knowledge and teaching methods for IPL facilitation. The final themes were the result of much discussion with the team and revisiting the data on a number of occasions. The final results were then organised into five main themes.

Sample

Acknowledging the limitations of this method, great care was given to the process of selecting the expert panel and providing feedback to them before the subsequent round. The study relied on purposive sampling, the researcher selecting the expert panel based upon strict criteria to ensure reliability. The criteria were circulated (Box A2.1) to the project steering group and two professional bodies within health and social care, CAIPE (Centre for the Advancement for Interprofessional Education) and LTSN (Learning and Teaching Support Network). Participants had to be recommended by their peers to ensure rigour, and the panel constituted a range of professional backgrounds to provide a genuine interprofessional nature.

As the research was a part of a larger project looking at the preparation of facilitators for interprofessional education, ethical approval was granted by the ethics committee at the University of Reading.

BOX A2.1 Criteria for selecting panel members

1 Has operational experience in the field of health and social care.
2 Holds professional or academic qualifications in health and/or social care.
3 Has worked as a facilitator with two or more different professional groups
4 Has at least two years experience of facilitating learning either within their own workplace or external workplace settings.
5 Has a good understanding of adult learning processes, through gaining a teaching qualification or learning acquired elsewhere.
6 Is able to meet learning objectives and targets set at the outset of a training session, measured through evaluation/assessment of the training session.
7 Has enthusiasm for and interest in their subject and can generate similar feelings for the subject in their students (the 'X' factor).
8 Is able to apply appropriate theory to explain and clarify practice.

Data collection

The research process was initiated using a questionnaire produced online for the participants (can be accessed online at www.pipe.ac.uk).[2] There were questions to ascertain quantitative information on professional background, training, etc. The majority of the questions were open ended to obtain data on the qualities thought to be necessary for effective facilitation. The questions aimed to identify differences in skills and knowledge between facilitation of uniprofessional groups and IPL groups. Care was taken in the planning and analysis of the questionnaire to overcome the bias that may be levelled at this method of data collection. The questionnaire used in the second round, structured according to the feedback and results from the first round, was similarly prepared and administered. Its principal aim was to establish consensus on the knowledge and skills necessary for the facilitation of interprofessional learning.

Data analysis

The process, using a grounded theory approach, required the use of three interrelated tasks to organise the information and identify patterns, develop ideas and then to draw on, verify and reach conclusions. The data was then examined to identify, code and categorise results, seeking emerging themes and concepts.[3] Cross tabulation analysis of the quantitative data to the qualitative data was undertaken as a means of identifying any correlative relationship between independent variables, such as experience, recent training, different areas of expertise, etc.

Finally, the themes emerging from the study were discussed with the scheme three team in an effort to minimise or eliminate researcher bias and thus ensure face validity. Whilst the systematic drawing together of information helped in the understanding of facilitation skills, discussions within the team underscored the need to acknowledge that this was not a value-free process. Self awareness was required to recognise the influence of the personal and professional knowledge and experiences of interprofessional teaching and learning. Triangulation was used to maintain a rigorous approach in the form of data collected from more than one geographical location, and data triangulation by referring data and interpretations back to the subjects, to reach a consensus on the skills necessary for the facilitation of IPL.

Results

Panel response

Of the 30 individuals identified for the expert panel, there was an overall response rate of 18. Although the response was initially disappointing, the respondents were representative of the professional mix and the panel consisted of doctors (including GPs), nurses, allied health professionals, teachers and managers. Despite having a number of social workers on the panel they unfortunately did not respond. At the time it was considered that around 30 participants would be sufficient. In hindsight, selecting a higher number in the beginning may have ensured more panel members, although according to Murray and Hammons there is little evidence that increasing the group size achieves any better result.[4] However, whilst it is recognised that this is a small scale study and is therefore not generalisable, it has provided important evidence on facilitation of work based IPL on which to base discussion and carry out further research.

The professional background of the respondents listed eight from a nursing background, five with a medical background, three allied health professionals, one teacher, and one National Health Service manager. Generally speaking, panel members facilitated groups of between 10 and 30 people, and the majority had over 10 years experience facilitating interprofessional learning. All the panellists had received training on adult learning processes but, despite this, three out of four claimed they had gained their facilitation skills mainly through experience; 55% had a professional teaching qualification, and a further 44% had attended short courses and study days. The cross tabulation analysis for the question on professional background provided some interesting results: for instance, six of the eight nurses had a professional teaching qualification, whereas only one of the five doctors fell into this category, the latter tending towards attendance of short courses and gaining skills through experience. The panel identified a wide range of groups they had facilitated including voluntary services, paramedics, fire services, schools, primary healthcare teams, and groups in hospitals, for example, accident and emergency staff.

Findings

At the start of the project and during the preparation of the questionnaire a number of important qualities necessary to be an effective facilitator were identified by the PIPE team and from the literature available on group facilitation. During the first round analysis of the findings it was decided to take the five highest percentage qualities for facilitation of interprofessional groups that the expert panel had prioritised as important:
- ability to establish relationships (83%)
- aware of diversity (60%)
- knowledge of adult learning principles (50%)
- ability to be reflective (45%)
- ability to be flexible (41%).

The results were distributed to the panel and the second questionnaire prepared and structured around the above qualities, incorporating wherever possible direct quotes from the first round (www.pipe.ac.uk).[2] Panel members were given the results of their colleagues' ranking of the qualities deemed as important for effective facilitation of IPL from the initial round and asked them to reconsider their views in the light of the findings. The aim of the second round was to gain a consensus on the teaching methods and skills necessary for facilitation of IPL, with the panel having the benefit of the results from the first round.

Following the analysis of the second questionnaire, the final outcomes of the results demonstrated that to prepare facilitators for IPL they need to acquire advanced and in-depth skills of facilitation, similar to those required to facilitate other complex diverse groups. But more importantly the results produced some very rich data about the sort of skills, knowledge and teaching methods for IPL facilitation. The final themes were the result of much discussion with the scheme three team and revisiting the data on a number of occasions. The team were divided into pairs and each asked to take one area to objectively explore thoroughly. The final results were then organised into five main themes. These can be seen in Chapter 3 where the findings of the study are discussed and related to interprofessional learning in practice.

APPENDIX 3

PIPE two research process using the Radnor framework

KATY NEWELL-JONES

The PIPE two project consisted of two phases. Phase I involved a process of collaborative engagement between members of each of the programme teams to share expertise and strengthen the IPL component of their respective postgraduate programmes in learning and teaching. Phase II consisted of a series of focus groups involving programme teams and students from the postgraduate learning and teaching programmes in each of the four HEIs. These focus groups discussed the underpinning values and challenges of IPL, the factors which in their opinion promoted and inhibited effective IPL practice and some of the outcomes which they have experienced. The data from the focus groups was analysed using Radnor's[1] framework for interpretive research in educational settings, resulting in the identification of recommendations for incorporating IPL into postgraduate programmes in learning and teaching. There was an additional data set collected through scheme two of curriculum developments and institutional changes which are explored in Chapter 6.[2]

Research methodology and methods

In January 2003, at the beginning of the PIPE project, the broad research question for scheme two was, 'how can IPL most effectively be incorporated into postgraduate teaching programmes?' Initial discussions explored both positivist and interpretive research approaches.

The field of IPL is complex with few definitive answers. There was an attraction towards identifying clear-cut solutions to straightforward questions through a positivist approach utilising experimental designs and a hypothetico-deductive process.[3]

It might have been possible to have adopted different modes of programme delivery at each of the four different HEIs, to have carried out a comparative analysis and to have arrived at definitive answers to the questions we were asking ourselves at the time. For example:

- is IPL most effectively embedded into a programme when it is explicitly addressed in discrete modules which students encounter at the beginning of their programmes, or where IPL is embedded in more subtle ways across the entire programme? Or are both required for maximum impact on the practice of participants?

- is an interprofessional cohort an essential component of developing IPL practices? If so what does that interprofessional cohort look like?

This approach was rejected for a number of reasons. Firstly, there were an enormous number of variables between the different programmes including the interprofessional nature of the cohort, the experience of the teaching teams, the existing structure and focus of the programmes to mention just a few. With a sample size of four, it would have been extremely difficult to make reliable causal links between modes or characteristics of delivery and outcomes. Secondly, and perhaps more importantly, the questions which we, as a research team, were asking were evolving as a result of our engagement in the project and deepening in our own understanding of IPL. Thirdly, the scheme consisted of four masters level programmes, each with teaching teams immersed to differing degrees in IPL and more than 150 health and social care professionals who were students on the programmes and actively engaged in studying learning and teaching in relation to their own complex interprofessional contexts. Some students on the programmes were active members of the PIPE student panel, attended conferences and workshops on IPL and were on the expert panel for the Delphi study.[4] Not only would it be difficult for PIPE scheme two members, who were also programme team members, to be objective researchers into the processes taking place in our own institutions, we would also miss the opportunity to draw on the wealth of experience within the programmes.

In her work on interpretive educational research, Radnor[1] described the process of the researcher making sense by understanding the complexity through the people who are actively involved in the challenges and issues under investigation. As members of programme teams, we were engaged with these challenges. We also had access, in the form of the students on the programmes, to a considerable pool of experience of health and social care professionals engaged in IPL as practitioners and as educators. This led to the decision to immerse ourselves fully within the process of enquiry as participant-researchers through a structured, interpretive research.

Pole and Lampard[5] recognise the value in a flexible and adaptive research design for qualitative research, which takes into account new learning and unanticipated events. This was certainly the case for phase I of our research, where the programmes in each of the HEIs were being adapted through a collaborative process. However, the data collection and analysis were designed to be highly structured and iterative.

The study design is explained following the aspects described by Lewis[6] in relation to qualitative research design.

Defining the research question

The research question was:

> What are the key factors in promoting IPL in postgraduate programmes in teaching and learning?

The purpose behind promoting IPL was to support the development of lecturers and practice educators, able and willing to identify and use interprofessional opportunities for collaborative learning, with the intention of positively promoting interprofessional working practices.

Populations and samples

The study drew on the active engagement of the programme teams and students on the postgraduate programmes in learning and teaching at each of the four HEIs during the period 2003–2005. All members of programme teams and all students were invited to participate. All those who responded positively were invited to participate in the focus groups which were held at set times. Sampling therefore was purposeful and depended on availability and interest. Programme team focus groups were separate from student focus groups.

The programme teams consisted of experienced educators and practice educators, from nursing, education, midwifery, occupational therapy, social work, science, podiatry, speech and language therapy and human resource management. In each of the four focus groups for programme teams there were between four and eight participants, which consisted of the majority of the core programme team.

At BCUC the students on the MA education (Nursing, Midwifery and Health Visiting) programme were primarily nurses with representation from midwifery and health visiting. At OBU the students on the MSc Higher Professional Education programme were primarily nurses (adult nursing, mental health, children's, community, palliative care) with representation from midwifery, occupational therapy, physiotherapy, medicine (general practice), social work, radiography, podiatry, dietetics, health careers advisory service and teenage pregnancy advisory service. At UR the students on the MA education (Health and Social Care) were primarily nurses with representation from podiatry, radiography, medicine and social work. At TVU the students on MA Learning and Teaching were nurses and midwives until 2004 when the programme was offered across the university and human resource management students joined the programme. In each of the focus groups there were between 4 and 10 participants from a cohorts of between 14 and 36 students.

Negotiation of research relationships and ethics

The research relationships in this project were complex and required specific consideration in order to avoid coercion and minimise the impact of researcher bias in the data collection and analysis. The scheme team were members, and in some instances leaders, of the MSc/MA programme teams in their respective institutions. Gold (1958, cited in Radnor)[1] described four stances which researchers can take in social science research:

- complete observer
- observer as participant

- participant as observer
- full participant.

The first is not possible in interpretive research and certainly not in this instance with the level of awareness and involvement of the research team. All students involved in the study were full participants as were most members of the programme teams. However, different stances were taken by the scheme team at different phases of the study. Great care was taken to discuss these differences, the tensions they might bring, and the measures required to reduce bias.

During phase I the scheme team were engaged in collaborative learning which resulted in changes in the ways in which IPL were incorporated into the programmes. At this stage the scheme team were 'participants as observers', i.e. engaged primarily in the process of enhancing the IPL aspect of the programmes, but also aware of the inter-institutional relationships and the overarching aim of the study. A high level of trust and depth of critical enquiry was established during this phase which enabled peer critique and sharing of challenges and potential strategies.

For phase II, an experienced researcher was brought into the team to facilitate the focus groups, who had not been involved in the scheme until that point and had no direct involvement in any of the learning and teaching modules on the MSc/MA programmes. She adopted the role of observer as participant. This enabled the members of the PIPE scheme to be full participants in the focus groups. Initially there was a fear that PIPE scheme members would be unable to detach themselves from the overall aim of the project, however, each found that having the focus groups facilitated by an independent experienced researcher, enabled them to focus on their role as a member of the programme team.

The data analysis was undertaken as a collaborative activity by the PIPE scheme team, together with the focus group facilitator and two additional programme team members who were new to the scheme. This gave a balance of observers as participants and participants as observers.

The research project was approved through the research protocol at the University of Reading and the Research Ethics Committee at Oxford Brookes University.

Timeframes for data collection
The focus groups took place over a period of three months between December 2004 and February 2005. This enabled all focus groups to be facilitated by the external researcher and also for the timing of the sessions to fit in with the availability of students and programme team members.

Data collection
Two kinds of data were collected. Firstly, descriptive information was gathered on the nature of the MSc/MA programmes at the beginning of the project and again

two years later. This enabled changes in the structure and content of the programmes, the constitution of the student cohort and the programme teams to be reviewed.

The main data set was from eight focus groups, two in each HEI, one consisting of members of the programme team and the other with students from the programme. Letters of invitation accompanied by an information sheet were sent to all students on the MSc/MA Education programmes who had been studying on the programme for at least six months. The focus groups were organised on days when core modules took place in order to minimise disruption and additional travel time for participants. Focus groups varied in size from four to ten. Letters of invitation, accompanied by the same information sheet, were sent to all members of programme teams who would usually be invited to attend programme review meetings. This included a number of people who were not involved in direct delivery but who supported students on their educational placements. In one institution there were difficulties with organising the student focus group and this was replaced by a questionnaire which students were invited to complete and return to the programme administrator.

The focus groups facilitated by the external researcher, were semi-structured in nature, lasted approximately one hour and were tape recorded.

Phase I – enhancing IPL in MSc/MA programmes

From January 2003 until December 2004 the PIPE scheme two team worked as a learning set, sharing experiences and exploring approaches to incorporating IPL into postgraduate learning and teaching programmes. The process was iterative and cyclical in nature, characterised by periods of collaborative engagement, deepening understanding, challenging assumptions and developing new initiatives. These were followed by developments in each HEI, the outcomes of which informed subsequent collaborative engagements.

The programmes began from different starting points and brought different experiences. Two institutions had been actively engaged in the Joint Universities Multiprofessional Progamme (JUMP) project previously,[7] another had a module in IPL which had been a core module since 2000. One programme was strengthening its links with the local Deanery, which is a partnership between the university medical school and the National Health Service (NHS) operating entirely within the NHS, with responsibility for providing education and training for doctors and dentists. As a consequence of this collaboration, General Practitioner trainees and trainers were accessing the MSc programme. Another of the institutions in scheme two was in the process of redesigning its MA Education programme as a generic teaching and learning programme offered across the HEI.

As a result of the collaborative activity it was agreed that each programme team needed to select the ways in which IPL was embedded in its programme and an acceptance that these needed to be different. However, there was also a need for consistency of approach, therefore from September 2003, all students on each of the programmes would explicitly 'explore opportunities for inter-professional collaboration which influence or lead to informal/formal learning'. This was achieved in different ways in each programme involving a combination of developing modules specifically exploring IPL, embedding learning outcomes relating to IPL into the core modules, and the inclusion of IPL in assessment tasks and marking criteria.

Data analysis

The focus groups were tape recorded and transcribed by an independent person who coded according to the institution and whether the participants were students or programme team members. Each individual contributor was also given a code. Scheme members worked from these coded transcripts in pairs of people from different HEIs to reduce institutional and individual bias.

Radnor's[1] framework for the analysis of interpretive research data in educational settings was adopted. Her process is systematic and she gives the rationale behind each of the stages, together with examples which enabled those new to interpretive research to gain insight into the process as a whole and each stage. Radnor[1] describes six specific steps in linear sequence. At first glance, it might appear that the steps are in contradiction to other interpretive frameworks for data analysis, as the first step is topic ordering, thus suggesting that the themes are selected from the first read. However, these topics are not the final themes for discussion, but are a means of holding the data in this interim period. The final categories emerge through a more in-depth and iterative process involving steps two to five.

Step 1 Topic ordering
Topic ordering was carried out as a whole group activity with pairs of team members from different institutions reading the eight transcripts and identifying key topics. These were shared and discussed within the team and a consensus emerged of six topics, drawn from across all the transcripts. It was interesting to note that the topics selected did not reflect those 'expected' from team members prior to the process. These moments of surprise were reassuring in that they indicated inductive processes were shaping the data analysis.

Step 2 Constructing categories
Categories were constructed under each of the topics through a process of immersion in the transcripts. Initially individuals identified both explicit and implicit categories which then underwent a peer review process. Each topic had between three and four categories, some of which were amalgamated in the review process.

Steps 3, 4 and 5 Reading for content; completing the coded sheets; generating coded transcripts
These steps took place as an iterative process where key quotes were identified, coded to topic categories, coding sheets were completed and specific quotations

were selected which typified each category. At the end of this stage the categories are confirmed and supported by coded sheets cross-referencing them to the transcripts and the transcripts are also coded.

Step 6 Analysis to interpretation of data

Finally, the team met to review the process and issues arising from the data analysis and the implications of the findings. Radnor[1] describes this as a refining process where meaning is drawn down from the data through an interpretive process. A position paper was produced summarising the three themes (*see* Chapter 4) which arose from the refining process together with their implications.

The findings to this study are presented and fully discussed in Chapter 4.

References

About this book

1 Illeris K. Towards a contemporary and comprehensive theory of learning. *Intern J Lifelong Educ.* 2003; **22**(4): 396–406.

CHAPTER 1 Perspectives of interprofessional learning and teaching

1 Miller C, Freeman M, Ross N. *Interprofessional Practice in Health and Social Care.* London: Arnold; 2001.

2 Freeth D, Reeves S. Learning to work together: using the presage, process, product (3P) model to highlight decisions and possibilities. *J Interprof Care.* 2004; **18**(1): 43–56.

3 Parsell G, Bligh J. Interprofessional education. *Postgrad Med J.* 1998; **74**: 89–95.

4 Atkins J. Tribalism, loss and grief: issues for multiprofessional education. *J Interprof Care.* 1998; **12**(3): 303–7.

5 Whittington C, Bell L. Learning for interprofessional and inter-agency practice in the new social work curriculum: evidence from an earlier research study. *J Interprof Care.* 2001; **15**(2): 158–67.

6 Barr H. *Interprofessional education: today, yesterday and tomorrow.* Occasional paper No 1 London: LTSN for Health Sciences and Practice; 2002.

7 Ewens AE. The changing role perceptions of students on integrated courses in community healthcare nursing. Unpublished PhD thesis. University of Reading; 1998.

8 Shakespeare H, Tucker W, Northover J. *Report of a national survey on interprofessional education in primary care.* London: CAIPE; 1989.

9 Howkins E, Thornton C, editors. *Managing and Leading Innovation in Health Care.* London: Bailliere Tindall; 2002.

10 World Health Organisation. *Learning Together to Work Together for Health.* Geneva: WHO; 1988.

11 Braithwaite J, Travaglia J. *Draft 2 Interprofessional Learning and Clinical Education: an overview of the literature.* Australia: Braithwaite and Associates; 2005.

12 CAIPE. *Interprofessional Education: a definition.* London: Centre for Advancement of Interprofessional Education; 2007.

13 Freeth D, Hammick M, Scott R, *et al. Effective Interprofessional Education: development, delivery and evaluation.* Oxford: Blackwell; 2005.

14 Department of Health. *The New NHS: modern and dependable.* London: DoH; 1997.

15 Department of Health. *A First Class Service: quality in the new NHS.* London; DoH; 1998.

16 Department of Health. *Working Together to Safeguard Children.* London: DoH; 1999.

17 Department of Health. *A Health Service of all the Talents: developing the NHS workforce. Consultation document on the review of workforce planning.* London: DoH; 2000.

18 Department of Health. *The NHS Improvement Plan.* London: DoH; 2004.

19 Drinka T, Tsukuda R. Conference Report for the Twenty-first Annual Interdisciplinary Healthcare Team Conference. *J Interprof Care.* 2000; **14**(2): 205–7.

20 Department of Health. *Learning for Collaborative Practice with Other Professions and Agencies.* London: DoH; 2003.

21 Department of Health. *Working Together to Safeguard Children: a guide to inter-agency working to safeguard and promote the welfare of children.* London: DoH; 2006.

22 Howkins E. Accepting the surfing challenge: making sense of collaboration. In: Howkins E, Thornton C, editors. *Managing and Leading Innovation in Health Care.* London: Bailliere Tindall; 2002.

23 Sullivan T. Concept analysis of collaboration: part 1. In: Sullivan T. *Collaboration: a health care imperative.* New York: McGraw-Hill; 1998; p 428.

24 Humphris D, Hean S. Educating the future workforce; building evidence about inter-professional learning. *J Health Serv Res Policy.* 2004; **9**(1): 24–7.

25 Tope R. *The Impact of Interprofessional Education in the South West Region: a critical analysis.* The literature review. London: DoH; 1998.

26 Barr H, Koppel I, Reeves S, *et al. Effective Interprofessional Education: argument, assumption and evidence.* London: CAIPE, Blackwell Publishing; 2005.

27 JUMP 2 North West London Workforce Development Confederation. *Evaluation report of Joint Universities Multiprofessional programme 2 2002–2004.* Programme supported by North west London Workforce Development Confederation; www.dh.gov.uk/policyandguidance

28 Reeves S, Freeth D, McCrorie P, *et al.* 'It teaches you what to expect in future...': inter-professional learning on a training ward for medical, nursing, occupational therapy and physiotherapy students. *Med Educ.* 2002; **36**: 337–44.

29 Mhalorunaigh S, Clifford C. The preparation of teachers for shared learning environments. *Nurs Educ Today.* 1998; **18**: 178–82.

30 Camsooksai J. The role of the lecturer practitioner in interprofessional education. *Nurs Educ Today.* 2002; **22**: 466–75.

31 Gilbert J, Camp R, Cole C, *et al.* Preparing students for interprofessional teamwork in healthcare. *J Interprof Care.* 2000; **14**(3): 223–5.

32 Barr H. Competent to collaborate: towards a competency-based model for interprofessional education. *J Interprof Care.* 1998; **12**(2): 181–8.

33 Schon D. *The Reflective Practitioner.* New York: Basic Books: 1983.

34 Schon D. *Educating the Reflective Practitioner.* San Francisco: Jossey-Bass; 1987.

35 Schon D. *The Reflective Practitioner: how professionals think in action.* Aldershot: Avebury; 1991.

36 Wee B. *Working together and learning together: a collaborative project.* Final report. Countess Mountbatten House and Moorgreen Hospital, Southampton; 1997.

37 Knowles MS. *The Adult Learner: a neglected species.* 4th ed. Houston: Gulf; 1990.

38 Howkins E, Allison A. Shared learning for primary healthcare teams: a success story. *Nurs Educ Today.* 1997; **17**(3): 225–31.

39 Fallesberg M, Hammar M. Strategies and focus at an integrated interprofessional training ward. *Med Teacher.* 2000; **21**(6): 576–81.

40 O'Halloran C, Hean S, Humphris D, *et al.* Developing common learning: the new generation project undergraduate curriculum model. *J Interprof Care.* 2006; **20**(1): 12–28.

41 Sarles H. *Teaching as Dialogue.* University Press of America; 1993 (out of print). Reproduced with permission in the Higher Education Academy Newsletter Autumn 2005; Issue 16. www.health.heacademy.ac.uk

42 Freire P. *Pedagogy of the Oppressed.* New revised ed. London: Penguin; 1996.

43 Freire P. *Education: the practice of freedom.* London: Writers and Readers; 1974.

44 Newell-Jones K. Whose reality counts? Lessons from Participatory Rural Appraisal (PRA)

for facilitators of interprofessional learning. In: Colyer H, Helme M, Jones I, editors. *The Theory-Practice Relationship in Interprofessional Education*. London: The Higher Education Academy: Health Sciences and Practice; 2005.

45 Illeris K. *The Three Dimensions of Learning*. 2nd ed. Frederiksberg: Roskilde University Press; 2004.

46 Lawlor M, Handley P. *The Creative Trainer*. New York: McGraw-Hill; 1996.

47 Bee F, Bee R. *Facilitation Skills*. London: Chartered Institute of Personnel and Development; 1998.

48 Hogan C. *Facilitating Empowerment: a handbook for facilitators, trainers and individuals*. London: Kogan Page; 2000.

49 Hunter D, Bailey A, Taylor B. *The Essence of Facilitation: being in action groups*. Auckland, New Zealand: Tandem Press; 1999.

50 Heron J. *The Complete Facilitators Handbook*. London: McGraw-Hill; 2000.

51 Heron J. *Group Facilitation*. London: Kogan Page; 1993.

CHAPTER 2 A learning and teaching framework for interprofessional learning

1 Vygotsky L. *Thought and Language*. Revised and edited by A Kozulin. Cambridge, Massachusetts: MIT; 1986; p 283. Cited by Jarvis P, Holford J, Griffin C. *The Theory and Practice of Learning*. London: Kogan Page; 1986, p 35.

2 Illeris K. *The Three Dimensions of Learning*. Frederiksberg: Roskilde University Press; 2002, p 118.

3 Illeris K. Towards a contemporary and comprehensive theory of learning. *Int J Lifelong Educ*. 2003; **22**(4): 396–406.

4 Illeris K. Adult education as experienced by the learners. *Int J Lifelong Educ*. 2003; **22**(1): 13–23.

5 Illeris K. Transformative learning in the perspective of a comprehensive learning theory. *J Transformative Educ*. 2004; **2**(2): 79–89.

6 Colyer H, Helme M, Jones I. Pragmatic approaches and the theory-practice relationship in interprofessional education. In: Colyer H, Helme M, Jones I, editors. *The Theory-Practice Relationship in Interprofessional Education*. London: The Higher Education Academy: Health Sciences and Practice; 2005, pp 14–20.

7 Newell-Jones K. Whose reality counts? Lessons from Participatory Rural Appraisal (PRA) for facilitators of interprofessional learning. In: Colyer H, Helme M, Jones I, editors. *The Theory-Practice Relationship in Interprofessional Education*. London: The Higher Education Academy: Health Sciences and Practice; 2005; pp 63–8.

8 Sterling S. *Sustainable Education: revisioning learning and change*. Totnes: Green Books; 2001.

9 Bulman C, Shutz S, editors. *Reflective Practice in Nursing*. 3rd ed. Oxford: Blackwell Publishing; 2005.

10 www.gp-training.net Aids to GP training: educational theory. Adult learning. http://www.gp-training.net/training/restrain.htm (accessed 21.07.06) 2006.

11 Payne S. *Teamwork in Multiprofessional Care*. Basingstoke: MacMillan Press; 2000, p 199.

12 Carpenter C, Hewstone M. Shared learning for doctors and social workers. *Br J Soc Work*. 1996; **26**: 239–57.

13 Pettigrew TF. Intergroup contact theory. *Annual Review Psychology*. 1998; **49**: 65–85.

14 Dickinson C, Carpenter J. Contact is not enough: an intergroup perspective on stereotypes and stereotype change in interprofessional education. In: Colyer H, Helme M, Jones I, editors. *The Theory-Practice Relationship in Interprofessional Education*. London: The Higher Education Academy: Health Sciences and Practice; 2005, pp 23–30.

15 Adams A. Theorising inter-professionalism. In: Colyer H, Helme M, Jones I, editors. *The Theory-Practice Relationship in Interprofessional Education*. London: The Higher Education Academy: Health Sciences and Practice; 2005, pp 31–7.

16 Whittington C. Interprofessional education and identity. In: Colyer H, Helme M, Jones I, editors. *The Theory-Practice Relationship in Interprofessional Education.* London: The Higher Education Academy: Health Sciences and Practice; 2005, pp 42–8.

17 Allport GW. *The Nature of Prejudice.* Reading MA: Addison Wesley; 1954. Cited in Dickinson C, Carpenter J; 2005.

18 Freire P. *The Pedagogy of the Oppressed.* Penguin: Harmondsworth; 1972.

19 Mezirow J. *Transformative Dimensions of Adult Learning.* San Francisco: Jossey-Bass; 1991.

CHAPTER 3 Interprofessional facilitation skills and knowledge: evidence from a Delphi research survey

1 Illeris K. *Three Dimensions of Learning.* Roskilde: Roskilde University Press; 2004.

2 The PIPE Project: further information about the research and other work within the project is available online. www.pipe.ac.uk

3 Department of Health. *Working Together to Safeguard Children. A guide to inter-agency working to safeguard and promote the welfare of children.* London: DoH; 2006.

4 Department of Health. *The NHS Improvement Plan: putting people at the heart of public services.* London: DoH; 2003.

5 Department of Health. *The New NHS: modern and dependable.* London: DoH; 1997.

6 Department of Health. *The NHS Improvement Plan.* London: DoH; 2004.

7 Department of Education for Skills. *Every Child Matters.* London: DfES; 2003.

8 Whittington C, Bell L. Learning for interprofessional and inter-agency practice in the new social work curriculum: evidence from an earlier research study. *J Interprof Care.* 2001; **15**(2): 153–70.

9 JET (Joint Evaluation Team) Review. Koppel I, Barr H, Reeves S, *et al.* Establishing a systematic approach to evaluating the effectiveness of interprofessional education. *Issues in Interdis Care.* 2001; **3**(1): 41–50.

10 Lupton C, Khan P. The role of health professionals in the UK child protection system: a literature review. *J Interprof Care.* 1998; **12**(2): 209–21.

11 Laming, Lord. *The Victoria Climbie Inquiry.* London: DoH; 2003.

12 Kennedy I. *The Bristol Inquiry.* The Health Summary, XV111 No 7–8 July–August 2001 from CAIPE Bulletin, No 21 Winter 2001–2002.

13 JUMP 2 North West London Workforce Development Confederation. *Evaluation Report of Joint Universities Multiprofessional programme 2 2002–2004.* Programme supported by North West London Workforce Development Confederation; www.dh.gov.uk/policyandguidance

14 Crotty M. The emerging role of the British nurse teacher in Project 2000 programmes: a Delphi survey. *J Advanc Nurs.* 1993; **18**: 150–7.

15 Schwarz R. *The Skilled Facilitator: practical wisdom for developing effective groups.* California: Jossey-Bass; 1994, chapter 1.

16 Helme M, Sills M. *LTSN Triple Project: proposals for developing and sustaining interprofessional education initiatives in health and social care.* Conference Paper; 2003. http://www.triple-ltsn.kcl.ac.uk

17 Barr H. *Interprofessional education: today, yesterday and tomorrow.* Occasional paper No 1. London: LTSN for Health Sciences and Practice; 2002.

18 Bandura A. Modelling theory: some traditions, trends and disputes. In: Parke R, editor. *Recent Trends in Social Learning Theory.* New York: Academic Press; 1972.

19 Knowles M. *Andragogy in Action: applying modern principles of adult learning.* London: Jossey-Bass; 1985.

20 Schon DA. *The Reflective Practitioner: how professionals think in action.* Aldershot: Avebury; 1991.

21 Parsell, G. Spalding R, Bligh J. Shared goals, shared learning: evaluation of a multiprofessional course for undergraduate students. *Med Educ.* 1998; **32**: 304–11.

22 Moss B. The use of large-group role-play techniques in social work education. *Soc Work Educ*. 2000; **19**(5): 471–83.

23 Robertson N. Opportunities and constraints of teamwork. *J Interprof Care*. 1999; **13**(3): 311–8.

24 Freeman M, Miller C, Ross N. The impact of individual philosophies of teamwork on multiprofessional practice and the implications for education. *J Interprof Care*. 2000; **14**(3): 237–47.

25 Lizzio A, Wilson K. Facilitating group beginnings part 1: a practice model. *Groupwork*. 2001; **13**(1): 6–30.

26 Bourne D. *Moving on from the Victoria Climbie Inquiry*. CAIPE Bulletin, No 23; Spring 2004.

27 Humphris D, Hean S. Educating the future workforce: building evidence about interprofessional learning. *J Health Serv Res and Policy*. 2004; **9**(1): 24–7.

28 Gilmartin J. Teachers' understanding of facilitation styles with student nurses. *Int J Nurs Stud*. 2001; **38**: 481–8.

CHAPTER 4 Embedding interprofessional learning in postgraduate programmes of learning and teaching

1   Radnor H. *Researching Your Professional Practice: doing interpretive research*. London: Oxford University Press; 2001.

2   Barr H. *Interprofessional Education: today, yesterday and tomorrow*. London: LTSN; 2002.

CHAPTER 5 Preparing facilitators for interprofessional learning

1   Heron J. *The Complete Facilitator's Handbook*. London: Kogan; 2003.

2   Elwyn G, Greenhalgh T, Macfarlane F. *A Guide to Small Groupwork in Healthcare, Management and Research*. Oxford: Radcliffe Medical Press; 2001.

3   Jaques D. *Learning in Groups: a handbook for improving groupwork*. London: Routledge Falmer; 2000.

4   Reynolds M. *Groupwork in Education and Training: ideas in practice*. London: Kogan Page; 1994.

5   Carr W. *For Education: towards critical educational inquiry*. Buckingham: Open University Press; 1995.

6   Hogan C. *Practical Facilitation: a toolkit of techniques*. London and Sterling: Kogan Page; 2003.

7   Schon D. *Educating the Reflective Practitioner: towards a new design for teaching and learning in the professions*. San Francisco: Jossey-Bass; 1987, p 22.

8   Jarvis P. Reflective practice and nursing. *Nurs Educ Today*. 1992; **12**(3): 174–81.

9   Goodman J. Reflection and teacher education: a case study and theroretical analysis. *Interchange*. 1984; **15**(3): 9–26.

10 Fish D, Coles C. *Developing Professional Judgement in Healthcare: Learning through the critical appreciation of practice*. Oxford: Butterworth-Heinemann; 1998.

11 Illeris K. *Three Dimensions of Learning*. 2nd ed. Frederiksberg: Roskilde University Press; 2004.

12 Bond M, Holland S. *Skills of Clinical Supervision for Nurses*. Buckingham: Open University Press; 1998.

13 Department of Health. *The NHS Knowledge and Skills Framework*. London: DoH; 2004.

CHAPTER 6 Curriculum development for interprofessional learning

1   Iwasiw C, Goldenberg D, Andrusyszyn M-A. *Curriculum Development in Nursing Education*. Sudbury, Massachusetts: Jones and Bartlett; 2005.

2   Kelly AV. *The Curriculum: theory and practice*. 5th ed. London: Sage; 2004.

3   Uys LR, Gwele NS. *Curriculum Development in Nursing – process and innovations*. London: Routledge; 2005.

4 Neary M. *Curriculum Studies in Post-Compulsory and Adult Education: a teacher's and student's study guide*. Cheltenham: Stanley Thornes; 2002.

5 Bradbeer J. *Evaluation of Curriculum Development in Higher Education*. Technical Report No 8. Portsmouth: University of Portsmouth; 1998.

6 Whittington C. Interprofessional education and identity. In: Colyer H, Helme M, Jones I, editors. *The Theory-Practice Relationship in Interprofessional Education*. London: The Higher Education Academy: Health Sciences and Practice; 2005, pp 42–8.

7 O'Halloran C, Hean S, Humphris D, *et al*. Developing common learning: the New Generation Project undergraduate curriculum model. *J Interprof Care*. 2006; **20**(1): 12–28.

8 Marks-Maran D, Young G. Interprofessional learning: context, meaning and technology. In: Carlisle C, Donovan T, Mercer D, editors. *Interprofessional Education: an agenda for healthcare professionals*. Salisbury: Quay Books; 2005, pp 141–53.

9 Church C, Shouldice J. *The Evaluation of Conflict Resolution Interventions: framing the state of play*. Londonderry, Northern Ireland: INCORE; International Conflict Research (University of Ulster and the United Nations University); 2002.

10 Pawson R, Tiley N. *Realistic Evaluation*. London: Sage; 1997.

11 Kirkpatrick D. *Evaluating Training Programmes: the four levels*. San Francisco: Barrett-Kjoehler; 1994.

12 Chambers R, Conway G. *Sustainable rural livelihoods: practical concepts for the 21st century*. Brighton: Institute of Development Studies (IDS) Discussion Paper 296; 1991. http://www.livelihoods.org/info/guidance_sheets_pdfs/section1.pdf (accessed June 2006).

13 Carney D. *Sustainable Livelihoods Approaches: progress and possibilities for change*. London: Department for International Development (DFID); 2002. http://www71.livelihoods.org/info/docs/SLA_Progress.pdf (accessed July 2006).

14 Soussan J, Blaikie P, Springate-Baginski O, *et al*. *A Model of Sustainable Livelihoods. Improving Policy-Livelihood Relationships in South Asia*. Briefing Note 3. York: Stockholm Environment Institute; 2003 accessed at http://www.york.ac.uk/inst/sei/prp/pdfdocs/3%20livelihoods%20factsheet.pdf (accessed July 2006).

15 Illeris K. *The Three Dimensions of Learning*. Frederiksberg: Roskilde University Press; 2002.

16 Jackson N. *Developing Creativity in Higher Education: the imaginative curriculum*. Abingdon: Routledge Falmer; 2006.

17 Barnett R, Coate K. *Engaging the Curriculum in Higher Education*. Buckingham: SRHE/Open University Press; 2004.

18 Stenhouse L. *An Introduction to Curriculum Research and Development*. London: Heinemann; 1975, p 199.

19 Lawton D. *Social Change: educational theory and curriculum planning*. London: University of London Press; 1973.

20 Dickinson C, Carpenter J. Contact is not enough: an intergroup perspective on stereotypes and stereotype change in interprofessional education. In: Colyer H, Helme M, Jones I, editors. *The Theory-Practice Relationship in Interprofessional Education*. London: The Higher Education Academy: Health Sciences and Practice; 2005, pp 23–30.

21 Nyatanga L. The archetypal roots of ethnocentrism In: Colyer H, Helme M, Jones I, editors. *The Theory-Practice Relationship in Interprofessional Education*. London: The Higher Education Academy: Health Sciences and Practice; 2005, pp 69–78.

22 Gibson P. Life and learning in further education: constructing the circumstantial curriculum. *J Further High Educ*. 2004; **28**(3): 333–46.

CHAPTER 7 Collaboration beyond champions

1 Barr H, Ross F. Mainstreaming interprofessional education in the United Kingdom: a position paper. *J Interprof Care*. 2006, **20**(2): 96–104.

2 Barker K, Bosco C, Oandasan I. Factors in implementing interprofessional education and

collaborative practice initiatives: findings from key informant interviews. *J Interprof Care.* 2005; **19**(1): 166–76.

3   Freeth D. Sustaining interprofessional collaboration. *J Interprof Care.* 2001; **15**: 37–46.

4   Illeris K. *The Three Dimensions of Learning.* 2nd ed. Frederiksberg: Roskilde University Press; 2004, p 89.

5   Foucault M. *The Will to Knowledge: the history of sexuality.* Volume 1. Hurley R, translator. London: Penguin; 1998.

6   Iwasiw C, Goldenberg D, Andrusyszyn M-A. *Curriculum Development in Nursing Education.* Sudbury, Massachusetts: Jones and Bartlett Publishers; 2005.

7   Ginsberg L, Tregunno D. New approaches to interprofessional education and collaborative practice: lessons from the organizational change literature. *J Interprof Care.* 2005; **19**(1): 177–87.

8   Gilbert J. Interprofessional learning and higher education structural barriers. *J Interprof Care.* 2005; **19**(1): 87–106.

CHAPTER 8 Through the PIPE

1   Ross F, Barr H. Editorial. *J Interprof Care.* 2006; **20**(3): 223–4.

2   Hughes L, Marsh T, Lamb B. *Report of the working groups.* Creating an Interprofessional Workforce (CIPW); 2006. www.cipw.org.uk

3   Barr H, Ross F. Mainstreaming interprofessional education: a position paper. *J Interprof Care.* 2006; **20**(3): 96–104.

4   JUMP 2 North West London Workforce Development Confederation. *Evaluation report of Joint Universities Multiprofessional Programme 2, 2002–2004.* Programme supported by North West London Workforce Development Confederation. www.dh.gov.uk/policyandguidance

5   Humphris D, Hean S. Educating the workforce: building the evidence about interprofessional learning. *J Health Serv Res Policy.* 2004; **9**: 356–4.

6   Department of Health. *National Service Frameworks for Older People.* London: DoH; 2001.

7   Meads G, Ashcroft J. *The Case for Interprofessional Collaboration in Health and Social Care.* London: Blackwells; 2005.

APPENDIX 1 The PIPE project

1   Radnor H. *Researching Your Professional Practice: doing interpretive research.* London: Oxford University Press; 2001.

2   PIPE project. Final report; 2006. www.pipe.ac.uk

APPENDIX 2 PIPE three research methodology and methods

1   Crotty M. The emerging role of the British nurse teacher in Project 2000 programmes: a Delphi survey. *J Advanced Nursing.* 1993; **18**: 150–7.

2   The PIPE project. Further information about the research and other work within the project is available online: www.pipe.ac.uk

3   Polit F, Beck C, Hungler B. *Essentials of Nursing Research, Methods, Appraisal and Utilization.* 5th ed. Philadelphia: Lippincott, Williams and Wilkins; 2001, pp 329–33.

4   Murray JW, Hammons JO. Delphi: a versatile methodology for conducting qualitative research. *Review of Higher Education.* 1995; **18**: 423–36.

APPENDIX 3 PIPE two research process using the Radnor framework

1   Radnor H. *Researching Your Professional Practice: doing interpretive research.* London: Oxford University Press; 2001.

2   Lord M, Young G. Curriculum development. In: Howkins E, Bray J, editors. *Preparing for Interprofessional Teaching: theory and practice.* Oxford: Radcliffe Publishing; 2008, Chapter 6.

3 Parahoo A. *Nursing Research Principles, Processes and Issues*. Hampshire: Palgrave; 1997.

4 Bray J. Interprofessional facilitation skills and knowledge: evidence from a Delphi research survey. In: Howkins E, Bray J, editors. *Preparing for Interprofessional Teaching: theory and practice*. Oxford: Radcliffe Publishing; 2008, Chapter 3.

5 Pole C, Lampard R. *Practical Social Investigation: qualitative and quantitative methods in social research*. Harlow: Pearson Education; 2002.

6 Lewis J. Design issues. In: Richie J, Lewis J, editors. *Qualitative Research Practice: a guide for social science students and researchers*. London: Sage; 2003.

7 JUMP 2 North West London Development Confederation. *Evaluation report of the Joint Universities Multiprofessional Programme 2, 2002–2004*. Programme supported by North West London Workforce Development Confederation. www.dh.gov.uk/policyandguidance

Index